I0104593

The Twelve Principles of Light

The

Twelve Principles of Light

Healing for a Modern World

Dr. Millie Saha
MBBS MRCGP MFHom DRCOG
Licensed associate Pranic Healer

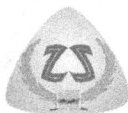

ZAMBEZI PUBLISHING LTD

Published in 2008 by
Zambezi Publishing Ltd
P.O. Box 221 Plymouth, Devon PL2 2YJ (UK)
web: www.zampub.com email: info@zampub.com

Copyright- text and front cover logo: © 2008 Millie Saha
Photographs © 2008 Jeremy Pounder
Cover design: © 2008 Jan Budkowski
Millie Saha has asserted the moral right
to be identified as the author of this work in terms of
the Copyright, Designs and Patents Act 1988

British Library Cataloguing-in-Publication Data:
A catalogue record for this book is available from
the British Library

Typeset by Zambezi Publishing Ltd, Plymouth UK
Printed and bound in the UK by Lightning Source (UK) Ltd

(ISBN-13): 978-1-903065-67-9

135798642

All rights reserved. No part of this publication may be reproduced, stored in a retrieval system, or transmitted in any form or by any means, electronic, mechanical, photocopying, recording, digital or otherwise, without the prior written permission of the publisher.

This book is sold subject to the condition that it shall not, by way of trade or otherwise, be lent, resold, hired out, reproduced or otherwise circulated, without the publisher's prior written consent or under restricted licence issued by the Copyright Licensing Agency Ltd, London, fully or partially, in any binding, cover or format other than in which it is originally published, and without a similar condition being imposed on the subsequent purchaser.

No warranties, either express or implied, are made by the author or the publisher regarding the contents of this book. The intention is to provide general information regarding the subject matter, and neither the author or publisher shall have any responsibility to any person or entity regarding any loss or damage caused or alleged to be caused, directly or indirectly, by the use or misuse of information contained in this book. If you do not wish to be bound by the above, you may return this book in good condition to the publisher for a full purchase price refund.

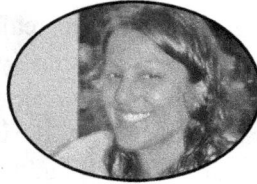

About the Author

Dr Millie Saha is a holistic GP and Integrated medicine specialist, currently based in London. She works within the NHS as full time GP, and in her private practice Fusion Medicine, based in Harley Street. Writing from her experience as a medical visionary and as a mirror of her quest to enlighten, teach and cure, Millie is dedicated to expanding our view of world spirituality as a path to greater personal health and global awakening.

She graduated from Kings College School of Medicine and Dentistry in 1996 and qualified as a GP, gaining membership in 1999.

During this time, Millie developed a keen interest in complementary medicine and alternative ways of managing illness. She completed medical homeopathy training to membership level through the Royal London Homeopathic Hospital, Great Ormond Street.

She remains committed to expanding our concepts of well-being and disease. She has had a natural ability to sense and intuit health through the energy body for many years, but condensed her knowledge by studying Pranic Healing whilst living in Sydney, Australia. She became a Licensed Associate Pranic Healer in 2003.

Millie is involved in bringing Integrated Medicine to the forefront of healthcare today, and is a GP associate on the Steering Group for the Prince's Foundation for Integrated Health. She also sits on the Committee for Complementary and Alternative Medicine at the Royal College of Physicians, and has been selected to practise Fusion Medicine at the renowned Hale Clinic in London.

Millie has a strong belief that, to really create health, you need to look far beyond the presenting symptom. To diagnose with the information held in the energy body and psyche alongside the physical, is to reveal the truth behind an illness. She believes that the key to healing the human body is to rebalance from within, integrating the best of all therapies to treat the mind, body and spirit.

She continues to offer a service that is bound to the principles of respect, honesty and compassion.

Millie lives in London with her husband Jez, daughter Clara and English Springer Spaniel Jimmy. She loves to travel and has spent time in South America, Australia and New Zealand, South Africa, Thailand and all over Europe.

She also loves writing, reading modern literature, walking the dog, watching movies and interior design.

Further information and Millie Saha's contact details are available from *www.fusionmedicine.co.uk*

For Jez, Clara and Jimmy; for showing me heaven...
Thanks,
Millie

Contents

The Journey into Light   3

Introduction   5

PART I   17

The Twelve Principles of Light   19

  1 Protection   21

  2 Abundance   35

  3 Creativity   51

  4 Trust   67

  5 Love   81

  6 Truth   95

  7 Wisdom   107

  8 Surrender   125

PART II   137

The Higher Soul Collective   138

  9 Peace   139

10 Karma   147

11 Forgiveness   155

12 Unity   165

Epilogue   173

Appendix   174

List of Therapists and Resources   176

Index   181

The Journey into Light

I have written The Twelve Principles of Light as a direct result of my calling to initiate, to educate, to heal and to love. The prophecy of truth spans generations but it has never been more important than now that we heed our true soul purpose in this new dimension. I hope the spiritual wisdom passed to me by my guides, to be chronicled in this book, may help you on your individual path to enlightenment.

As powerful free souls, we may achieve much, but as united world energy, we can achieve miracles. Our beloved planet is standing at the brink of a divine revolution; we alone are responsible for heralding a golden era of compassion, forgiveness, temperance and brotherhood.

Be brave and be wise, my friends.
Look to the light and find acceptance in your darkness.
This is a time for new ways.
This is a time for new beginnings.
This is a new dawn.
Fight like a warrior for our world.
Remember who you are.
Feel love.
Feel wisdom.
Feel faith.

Introduction

This is a book to open doors for you.

This is a book to make grand changes in the way you view your life and the way you view your world. We are living in dynamic, exciting and breathtaking times that move so fast that sometimes, if you stop for a second, it feels like you're lost in motion.

This is a book for everyone: for any age, time or place in your life when you seek hope, direction, solace or guidance.

The journey into light is an ongoing path that has led me from darkness into light, and I wish that you should also share it. What we aim to transform is not the exterior landscape but the vision within us. Look inwards, not outwards, because if we discover the beauty that we all hold deep inside we will be able to perform alchemy; our lives will turn to gold before our eyes.

I am hoping to reach those of you who have quietly asked: Is there more? How can I grow? How can I live my life in its fullest expression and make every second count? There is no set recipe for success as each of us is glorious in our individuality. To aspire to the heights is not to look at the standards set by others but to reach a point where we capture our very essence and set it free. We all have our grace and our given gifts, and to nurture these is to foster a future which allows us to shine. The grand design behind this is that we can not only flow freely but, in our happiness, extend to others the peace and kindness of our hearts. Love for ourselves becomes love for others and peace for humanity.

It seems simple, but if we could only illuminate the divinity in our own souls and be truly at peace with what we have and who we are, the darkness will not vanish but will instead cast contours and relief and enhance the brilliant light that each and every one of us holds.

Why should we travel – surely everyone wants only to feel peace of mind, happiness and love?

It is a cynical thing to look on life as an unhappy state – we are here to free our mind and soul and to run with the wind. We capture little pieces of time as our own to sail on and charge with momentum. Running requires discipline and strength, otherwise how do we protect ourselves should we stumble and fall? It takes practice, which is what the Principles are here to teach you. They will show you how to shine light onto shadow and how to stand still when all around you is in perpetual motion.

I work as a holistic general practitioner and vibrational energy healer, having initially trained as a medical doctor, graduating in 1996. Over the years I have had a chance to study the many faces of illness and disease but never as closely as when I am intuiting the energy system of my patient. The parallels that run between spiritual teachings and the evolution of our health system are amazing and seemingly unbelievable. It was through dealing with the transition from illness to health at each of the energetic levels that I began to see how, as we move towards health, our world vision shifts from the blocked or distorted to the truly enlightened.

We all suffer. We all experience difficulty and hardship on our way. We can all smile and laugh and love. What is often hard is finding a way to overcome our heartache. When there are no signposts it appears that only faith will bring salvation in our darkest hour. Through my discovery of the wonders of the energy body I believe it is possible to access the truth behind illness and disease and, by a process of working with our vibration, enable transformation to a higher state. The passage of healing is always a great lesson for the healed and the healer, as it brings both in touch with the divine. I am humbled by the channel of words through me that brings light to the sick and frightened, and helps me tend to those who have carried so much for so long. Healing takes courage and it requires making difficult decisions, but as we move towards our own personal truth, so our energy is freed. I see so many people turning emotional pain inwards, battling with memories of shame, neglect, self-loathing and bitterness, too paralysed to confront the darkness that lies within. With guidance and solid support we can all make changes of fate and lead a richer existence. Each illness comes with its own message; whether we listen and grieve and grow with it is our choice. It is always our choice.

~   So rise up, are you willing to heal?
~   I can help you now.
~   I can show you the way.

Follow with hope and faith and the Twelve Principles will deliver you to a new beginning. Your regret and sadness will be released with love and you can wake up to a new day of endless possibility.

The Meaning of Illness

I like to think of illness as a messenger. It usually alerts us to the fact that something within is not right and needs attention or rebalancing. Our physical bodies are infinitely wise and usually signal a need for soul expansion by using illness as a challenge to growth. In my experience an illness is seldom just a 'one symptom, one treatment' affair, but a multi-layered and complex picture. Each individual may present a different set of signs and complaints particular to his being. As a detective searches for clues, so the physician and healer will search the body for the ailment and create a diagnosis from what he finds.

The art of the search is to dig deep, and to think methodically and logically as well as to trust your intuition. As practitioners, our intuition is one of our most valuable tools and is often honed after seeing quite literally thousands of patients and building up in our subconscious a library of human disease. A cornucopia of information lies in the presentation, not only from the appearance, manner, history and examination of the physical body, but also from the energy body. It is possible to visualize a wealth of history from the hidden treasures in the blocked or damaged field.

Our illness lies bare but often we cannot see the truth. Our harmonic vibrations are unsettled, so how can we reset the pitch? The right person at the right time will set the wheels of healing in motion by acting as a catalyst on that person's path.

Vibrations

We all have vibrations. Every living being on this planet, every plant, mineral and animal has its own wavelength. The science of matter dictates that our molecular structure is in constant motion. We are growing and dying and changing and evolving every second. Although we exist as an energy system invisible to the naked eye, intuitive viewing makes the human field accessible to vision and touch and it is far more beautiful than you could ever imagine. In my mind's eye, I am blessed in clearly visualizing how wondrous the energy field can be when it is glowing with vitality and love. I see colours in every shade imaginable, cloudbursts of emotion and rapture, buried secrets, childhood fears, happiness, peace and unconditional love, the true desires of the soul.

Every thought, every feeling and every wish we have sings from us as a vibration. If we think something negative about others or ourselves this also impacts on our field or is picked up as a subtle subconscious vibration by our target. We know what we know. Our vibrations can transform others – we can affect change just by being. A child nurtured with loving thoughts grows up strong and secure; a child imprinted with negativity or poor messages finds it hard to thrive. So it is with the people around us; our positive thinking or negativity has an effect on our surrounding environment and can shape our experience of living. We have a responsibility in our actions – it is our free will to live our lives as we wish, but if we knew we could make a difference just by being, would we change?

We have one world connectivity; we have a universal soul, let us raise our consciousness together.

~ Love is the source.
~ Love is the transformation.
~ Love is always the heart and the answer.

The Chakras

Throughout this book I often mention the chakras, which are an integral part of our energy system. Chakras are whirling vortices of light, which extend from the human body and are palpable to the sensitized hand. There are over a hundred, varying in size, but the major ones are entitled Root, Sacral, Solar Plexus, Heart, Throat, Ajna, Forehead and Crown. There is also a spiritual cord that extends above the head and upwards, which is our connection to the divine. Each holds an emotional or mental key, a colour, a connection to the physical body and a developmental age. When each chakra is healthy it shines with a bright colour and a heightened energy of lightness, clarity and sweetness.

When a chakra becomes blocked, due to developmental, emotional or disease-related trauma, it will express lower levels of energy, or will be almost redundant, unable to express much at all. The chakra may appear tattered and empty and the patient often feels this way too. My job as a healer is to find out what hidden messages are buried in the field, to catalyze the release of pain and to implement the healing and mending of the energy system. My aim in this is to allow the patient to transcend his illness, to learn about and understand what his body has been trying to teach him, and to move towards a richer, better and healthier future. To live with perception and love is to live a deepened existence. We begin to live on earth as it is in heaven. We understand the spiritual principles through the very act of living and our beings express the wonder of spiritual bliss.

Releasing Pain

What happens when you release pain? Where does it go, what happens when it leaves? To see pain as a healer sees it is to see a black rain cloud, hovering like a dark mist over areas of the body. It appears as sludge, blackness or dirty energy, clogging up the field, preventing the colour and the light shining from the healthy body. Strip away the top layers and what you often see is the red raw pain of the trauma, a bleeding energetic injury. It is common also to sense the emotions behind this wound, the anger, rage and misery as well as the darts of negative thought and fear flowing in the darkness. People come to be healed when their souls tell them it is time to release and bid goodbye. It's been too long and the weight has been too heavy. The time to shed those self-destructive ways is when things have just started looking up, or when things have got so bad that the status quo cannot continue.

Working with the subtle vibrations through healing or flower essences, homeopathy or crystals helps release the old energy and leaves the patient ready to replace it with the new. Tears may accompany the loss of such an old companion; a false but faithful friend. A grief reaction tends to occur at the time of release as this grief was not expressed at the moment of truth; the sadness was suppressed at the bottom of the soul and a lid snapped tight until the right time came for clearing. The lid looks often like sealing wax or sticky glue; the conscious mind has willed it so that the pain is pushed down, never to see the light of day. At the time when events are fresh in the mind, the absence of examination gives temporary relief; a brief respite from seeing or feeling too much. But it is only temporary.

When something so heavy, and at odds with the true light nature, enters your body, you don't feel well. You may forget it's there, but it will play up. Pain is deceptive; it has many faces.

So next time you've taken self-destructive action, ask yourself what you are trying to escape from. What are you trying to diminish? Just be careful that the pain that you want some peace from doesn't take you down with it.

What is it that we are afraid of?
1. That which reflects the inner needs we deny ourselves.
2. That which makes us feel vulnerable.
3. That which triggers the pain body.
*4. That which reminds us of the parts of ourselves
that feel dis-ease.*
5. That which we don't understand.

~ From now on, learn to honour yourself, as we honour our world.
~ Release your pain body, as we release pain from our world.
~ Express yourself.
~ Protect yourself.
~ Accept yourself.
~ Educate yourself.

On this path to unity, remember compassion for yourself and others. Forgive yourself for your mistakes, as you forgive those who have trespassed against you. Travel light.

Integrated Medicine

I believe there is a place for all healing and medical modalities, but the best way is using integrated medicine as an individualized therapy, picking a collective of disciplines that will truly benefit in the gentlest way. Using medicine in this manner follows The Way – the path of least resistance. Illness needs us to understand and learn, to turn inwards and to listen quietly. Disease creates discord demanding deeper perception; a shift from the core base vibrations of resentment, fear, hatred, neglect, shame and lack of love to the higher forms of unconditional love, freedom from pain and personal power. When we heal we grow in stature, wisdom and strength. When we are governed by fear and ignore our true feelings we weaken and perish. Seek harmony and you will find peace. Harmony at all costs.

What we need for the future of universal health is a more honest approach to the way we heal our sick. We need an ethos of trust, respect and compassion to prevail; we need our healers to be committed to seeking truth in their own lives so their work becomes powerful and aligned with the higher vibrations of health our world now calls for. We need to put away our prejudices and fear of each other and work together for the common good.

It is a mighty gift to heal, as by the law of karma, that which you give you shall also receive. To give life is the elixir of immortality and lights the passage to unseen realms. It is a position to be honoured and treated with great responsibility. To heal without the vibration of love and respect is a lesser thing and surely something that detracts from the joy of interaction. In each unique healing connection, the energy of that moment will move towards the universal healing energy. We are going through such transitional times that the world soul will demand a higher level of understanding and spiritual intuition as we are pulled from one era to the next. More and more people are discovering the ability to sense the higher bodies, intuit energies in themselves and others, see the colours of an auric field and feel their own physical body lifting, becoming lighter and stronger.

Once this shift occurs on a personal level, the need for remedies and cures for treating the vibration are apparent and necessary. Homeopathy, flower essences, colour healing, energy healing, aromatherapy and crystal therapy are all excellent ways of shifting disease at a high vibrational frequency. Mind medicine, including hypnotherapy, NLP and psychotherapy are excellent at changing vibration through thought. Massage, acupuncture, kinesiology and bodywork physically work through multiple levels of the body and meridians and, finally, normal medicines and surgery are of vital necessity when administered with synchronicity and calling. Nothing can replace the miracles of modern medicine when that is what the body needs.

I think the future lies in a personalized integrated approach where the power is positioned with the sick person; his desire to be well drives the transformation from one life stage to another. As he heals, his spiritual unrest is resolved, his soul evolves by perception and his body is restored to balance.

How to Use This Book

This is a handbook of healing; it will give you comfort and solace on your journey into light and practical keys to ease open the locked doors of the mind. This book is suitable for anyone who is hoping to grow; to understand their life more deeply and move beyond the emotional and mental restrictions created in the psyche by challenging life experience. It is also for those who want to explore spiritually, open to the divine in everyday life, and become a stronger, calmer and more loving version of their original self. As a healer I work to clear the energy body of residual pain, to act as a catalyst for the soul to recognize the deep buried trauma and let it go once and for all. I work with people to realize their potential and beauty and allow them to be reborn. I want you to read this book and get it, get happy, wake up and see how wonderful you are, how much love and happiness you deserve and how to go about getting it. Try to stop going round in circles, stop fighting with yourself. Freedom comes with deep self-acceptance and refusing to conform to societal norms and expectations. Just be. After all, a happy person is at peace; his love shines out to the rest of us. The Principles will guide you there; the Principles are your teachers. Work with these masters and they will blaze the way.

Each chapter will have the lessons of the principle and selected exercises to work through. There will also be remedy stores detailed in the first eight principles, to enhance the healing process. These may be used according to the personal issues being raised. I have also added a few carefully chosen essences and crystals for the Higher Soul Collective. In all of this, I would like you to trust your intuition in finding your own path.

Take a month or so to absorb the teachings and practise each one of them until you own them, until you can hear them singing from your very self. Keep a special handbook or diary by your bed to record the changes as each month goes by. Make a note of what feelings and emotions arise and of how it feels to tend to yourself in this new way. Look at the pictures and let them inspire you. The beauty of the world is everywhere and reflects the beauty we also hide within. The photos were taken on a journey I took with my husband through South America, Australia, New Zealand and South Africa. It was a period of my life when everything was changing and I was leaving my past behind with every step I took into the future. Our earth opened my eyes and my soul with its power and continues to renew me as I ask of it. We are connected to the ground beneath our feet.

Ideally, write a journal entry every morning and evening - this is the process of paying attention and keeping your own counsel: a watchful waiting, growth through love and a record of the currents and tides that ebb and flow with your emotional health. The writing is a cleansing, an outpouring of the old as you welcome the new. It will also be your keepsake of dreams and desires.

If you are recommended to use vibrational remedies, homeopathy, crystals, aromatherapy or essences, ensure you follow the given instructions. Essences are usually taken two drops twice a day until there is a clear emotional shift, homeopathy as a 30c dose, once a day for three days. Essential oils can be used in a bath or as drops on your pillow; crystals must be soaked in salt water overnight and then charged by holding the crystal in your hands for ten minutes sending positive loving energy into it, asking the crystal to heal you. Crystals can be carried, worn or placed by your bed, but do not use crystal therapy if you are pregnant.

You will find more detailed instructions in the Appendix regarding the use of crystals. There are certain oils to avoid in pregnancy and these are also listed in the appendix, alongside a list of approved therapist sites and contact details.

I want you to sparkle with life.

The Principles follow your energy system from root to crown and beyond, but healing does not necessarily take place sequentially. Give yourself a bit more time in a particular area if you feel this is needed, or go back to it. You may encounter obstruction, hesitation, refusal, resistance. You may find the book gets left for day or weeks. It means something. When you come back to it, which I hope you will, ask yourself truthfully what happened. What was it that stopped you in your tracks? Did you stop because you were frightened? Did you feel pain? Did you decide to self-destruct a little because something was too hard to confront?

The journey carries us through muddy waters and faith is needed when emotion comes to the surface. Breathe and let it settle. Breathe and let it go. Breathe and in time all will pass. If you have courage the worst will be over and you will have moved on with deeper insight and greater self-respect; an understanding of who you are and what this is all about. Be brave. Each chapter will have the lessons of the Principle, a remedy store and a list of guides that may be relevant to the issues you face. In all of this I would like you to trust your intuition in finding your own path. Trusting your intuition will heighten the ease with which you move along your path. Do not force anything, just flow. Be gentle with yourself, have respect for yourself and take time every day to reconnect with your journey. Look to the light.

At the end of the tunnel lies truth, and beyond this lies infinite peace, with the acknowledgement that there is nothing buried or hidden any longer. You are free. Freedom can be frightening after years of institutionalized thinking. When there are no longer restrictions or limitations, the concept of doing whatever we want, whenever we want feels all too much. We can be whoever we choose to be, without judgement. There is, of course, no-one left to blame, there are no more excuses to be made. We are entirely responsible for our future destiny. We are faced with endless possibility. Will we live up to it and use our power wisely? There may be moments when you are scared and the truth is too much. This passage is all about willingness and if things speed up, slow a little, take a moment and affirm to yourself, 'I am willing'.' Look to the supports on your journey, those who commend you for seeking a greater life and provide safe shelter as you weather the storm.

At the end of the journey, you will find light, space, energy and the untapped potential of the divine soul. Do not be afraid of your brightness, your greatness. Rise to it and move towards it. Grow and become the person you always dreamed of. From the moment you were born, your soul has yearned for radiance. As we go through life, a split often occurs between our born self and our conditioned self; the person we were born to be and the person we are expected to be, or we think we should be. Now is the time to cut through those expectations and reunite with our true birthright, where just being is enough. Reclaim energy used in worrying about whether you are good enough, and channel it back into being the best you can be. Work with the journey into light, bringing you closer to yourself and bringing you home.

~ There is magic in transformation.
~ There is joy in reaching the top of the mountain.
~ There is peace in standing alone.
~ There is wisdom in learning from the path behind you.
~ There is courage in treading the path ahead of you.
~ There is grace in compassion.
~ There is power in creation.
~ There is love in acceptance.
~ There is freedom in forgiveness.
~ Journey with me.
~ Journey into light.

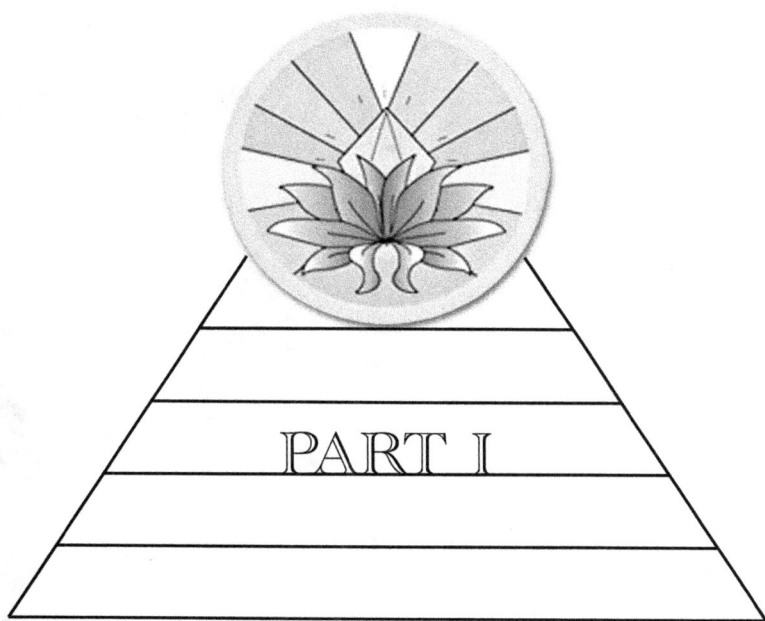

PART I

The
Twelve Principles of Light

1. Protection
2. Abundance
3. Creativity
4. Trust
5. Love
6. Truth
7. Wisdom
8. Surrender
9. Peace
10. Karma
11. Forgiveness
12. Unity

The Twelve Principles of Light are based on the major spiritual centres, and are deep core vibrations that we actualize and embody in our experience of existence. Each Principle connects to an energetic landmark in our development, and we travel from the root chakra to the crown chakra and beyond, as our consciousness is raised from the earthly plane to the ethereal. They are the height of soul evolution and the positive expression of man's humanity. They are what we are when we shine with the light of heaven.

~ The Principles will guide you.
~ The Principles will heal you.
~ The Principles will teach you.
~ The Principles will transform you.

Like a flame in the darkness, the Principles will blaze the Way.

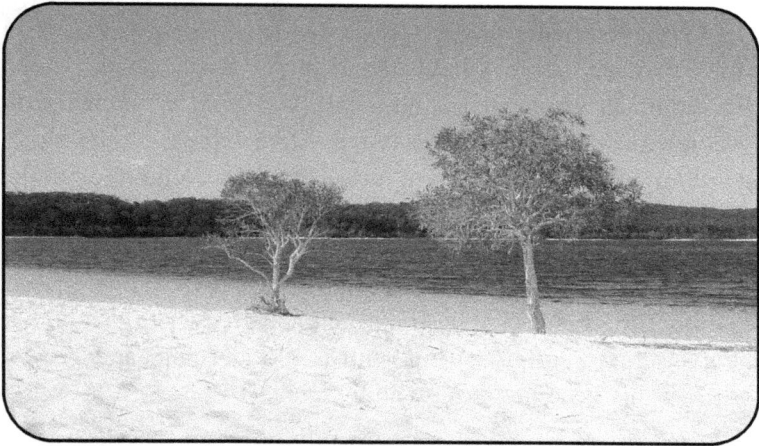

1

Protection

Protection greets us as the first of the Twelve Principles of Light.

Protection is the primary landmark in our spiritual journey – it is integral to the structure and stability of our being.

It is necessary to lay the foundations before you may build your castle. You could spend a lifetime nurturing happiness only to watch it washed away by the tides of life; we need to learn as warriors how to take steps to keep ourselves safe and dry. The universe asks you to consider carefully, watch wisely and be aware that to protect yourself is to consider yourself worthy and valuable. The message of this planetary vibration is one of grounding and security.

Protection is a balance between striking out into the world, fearless, feeling, thinking and relating as a humane, loving being and a perception of the real dangers and difficulties that lie ahead.

As a wild animal graces our eye with its beauty, it keeps a safe distance in the knowledge that not everyone has good intentions in that precise moment. We grow as humans to become most powerful in our true positive expression, living; to grow mighty we must prevent ourselves from colliding with the paths of those who may still be learning the values of integrity in the classroom of life.

We also need to protect ourselves from a myriad of elements in daily life, such as stress, pollution, negative energy and other people's toxic emotions, but with a strong shield and greater wisdom this becomes a more attainable task.

> *Protection opens our eyes to potential pitfalls and keeps the dark at our door.*
>
> *As you would protect a tiny child, so you should protect yourself.*
>
> *You are precious, vulnerable and priceless.*
>
> *The greatest protection in the world is the pure light of love.*

Protection is the first Principle, but is often the last to be taught.

Starting today, carry your protection and feel strong and sheltered as you undertake transformation.

Why Protection is Important

Protection is our defence system. It is the unseen fabric in every society that enables it to function smoothly and safely. It grants us the freedom as citizens to walk where we wish without fear or worry. On an individual level it enables us to go about our daily lives without interruption from the chaos that inevitably surrounds us. Healthy protection repels the negative energy of others and keeps us separate and detached. We know our own minds, remain resilient in the face of external pressure or control and truly shine in our soul expression.

Protection has never been more important than today, in our turbulent, challenging times. We cannot predict what dangers lie on our road ahead. All we can do is keep a clear head, enduring faith and knowledge of what we can do for ourselves.

Under the influence of others it is often hard to retain our individuality or make our own choices about life. I am sure you can picture a time when you were unclear whether the thoughts or feeling you had were your own or were being influenced by someone else. Can you remember a time when you picked up on the feelings or mood of those around you to the extent it made you feel as if you were carrying those emotions yourself? Protection does not dull your sensitivity; it merely acts as a necessary filter. This is even more important to those souls who have highly developed psychic and extrasensory powers. From this standpoint you gain distance and are more able to act with compassion. Right action is not coloured by the influence or will of a second party. Protection gives us dignity and a safe space; we are prevented from being dragged into another's drama and destiny and we retain our own energy to fire our own soul purpose and creativity.

Protection is freedom. We are able to express ourselves fully without the fear that we will not be accepted.

When we struggle with our own issues it is easy to project our shadow character onto others instead of taking ownership of those difficulties and working through them. For instance, if we are uncomfortable with our own need to control others we may see this quality in others easily and find it very difficult to deal with, instead of being able to see and accept ourselves for what we hold inside and move beyond it. Once we have dealt with it we are less likely to judge others as we no longer judge ourselves.

Our shield reflects any shadow projection back to its owner and we are more comfortable in shining brightly and standing out in a crowd. If we shrink to make others feel more comfortable in their insecurity and self-judgement all we succeed in doing is dishonouring our own divinity. In our protection we are immune to the thoughts and desires of others to shape us or mould us – we are free just to be.

Protection is most obviously important in preventing emotional and physical harm befalling us. It is essential in our journey through life and is intrinsic to our health and wellbeing as a developing soul. We have a responsibility to take precautions and measures to maintain a peaceful existence, just as in our world there are systems in place that prevent countless numbers of incidents occurring which could cause injury or damage to humanity. The defence systems in our society are always switched on, always on guard and ready to move at the slightest warning, and because of this we are able to live relatively untroubled lives. After witnessing random acts of terrorism or shattering natural disasters you may be forgiven for thinking that we should live our lives in fear; instead, focus on the life that is saved on a daily basis, the unseen forces at work every day that prevent untold accidents and fatalities.

As we learn to protect ourselves, practically and spiritually, we are building a future of sanctuary and safety. There will always be the unpredictable, the inevitable and the unavoidable, but to reduce the probability of ill fate we must practise our interventions and look ahead. In practical terms we are used to looking after our physical health, taking out insurance, making sure our car is serviced and our home is structurally sound. In spiritual terms, it is less understandable how we can be precautionary, but there are a few golden rules, which, if absorbed and respected, can give us an increased sense of faith and direction on our path.

How does Protection Develop?

Protection is a gift we are born into. Our earthly mother cloaks us in her protective energy field as we enter the world and we are dependent on her for our survival. As we grow, the love of our parents envelops us in warm security. The powerful light of unconditional love creates a tangible shield that is greater than the lower vibrations of fear and pain. We are inquisitive and joyful and carry light energy forward as incarnated souls; until the age of about seven these layers of protection give us the safety net to explore, play and grow into our individual personalities. This energy matrix is intrinsic to the young child.

In childhood we also learn certain patterns. We are taught to take care when crossing a road, not to go too close to a fire, not to talk to strangers – these are normal messages which are commonly handed down from adult to child. What can also leave a lasting effect on our innate ability to protect are the more personal imprinting and conditioning from our elders. This is all well and good if we are encouraged to explore and take care in equal measure, but what happens if parents are over-protective, or if children are not protected sufficiently?

An over-protected child's learning experience becomes limited, stifled and frustrated. He becomes unsure of himself when making choices and decisions. An element of fear is introduced. In later life these patterns may be played out as heightened anxiety and insecurity on multiple levels with the impulse to rebel or act out against authority or establishment. Ideals become confused and a young person may disregard the basic conventions of safety for the exhilaration of being free, or distrust his ability to manage or direct his own life successfully. A little protection well taught instils a healthy respect for the true dangers in the world but does not prevent active adventure or enjoyment of everything there is to offer.

When children are at risk, neglected or harmed, this lack of protection creates lasting damaging effects that must be healed. The memory of trauma is carried forward in the energy body and is overlaid on situations and relationships in later life. Until these imprints are understood and released they will engender difficulty in trusting and relating to others. These children grow up with the message that they were not valuable enough to be protected. This pattern continues and they often choose low self-esteem relationships or dynamics in the future that reiterate this inner belief. They also find it hard to define clear boundaries and may swing between being cold, wary and closed off, and pulling too close to people to derive the affection they crave, resulting in co-dependency or imbalanced dynamics.

In an ideal world all children are raised with unconditional love and support; this is enough to give them a healthy sense of security and self-worth.

~ Protection is a mirror of all that surrounds you.
~ Protection houses the spirit.
~ Protection seats you within your sanctuary walls.
~ Protection is the shell that wraps around our field, like the silver seventh layer, holding it all together.
~ Protection is value.
~ Protection is contentment.
~ Protection is peace.

The brighter the light, the greater the need for protection.

When Protection is Strong

~ We dance through life and we express ourselves in total honesty.
~ We are fearless yet aware.
~ We vibrate with love and trust but are mindful of the realities of life.
~ We stand upright and walk with dignity.
~ We speak our truth.
~ We are not afraid to live as the souls we were born to be.
~ We know our own mind and we act from the heart.
~ We remain unique and distinct in our separateness but extend friendship and compassion to humanity.
~ We have boundless energy but hold our power within, poised and intense.
~ We no longer please others to make our lives easier but believe in the value of standing up for our rights.

~ We are grounded and complete in our incarnation, experiencing each day as a new blessing, living each day in our true potential.

~ We feel strong enough to face the challenges in our path, we are brave enough to adventure and explore.

~ We know nothing is certain but have certainty that we are strong enough to cope with anything thrown our way.

~ We have healthy relationships and we remain steady in the face of confrontation or opposition.

~ We do not invite danger into our lives, we respect ourselves.

~ We value ourselves as children of the universe and move ever forward on our path to enlightenment.

~ We protect ourselves and the universe protects us in equal measures.

When Protection is Weak

~ We feel vulnerable and insecure.

~ We live in fear and find it difficult to rise to the call to grow.

~ We trust others and ourselves little.

~ We find it difficult to stand our ground and say no; we find it hard to maintain our boundaries.

~ We attract situations that reflect low protection in our field – theft, physical assault, emotional trauma, abusive relationships or self-destructive behaviour.

Protection is a measure of insight and deserving. We may have been raised with poor levels of protection and continue to accept less than we need. Insecurity is a normal sensation. It may take years before we realize, after a catalogue of bad experiences, that we need to change the very fabric of our existence. We may be unaware that we instigate the very scenarios that leave us feeling scared or frightened. The inner child that lives within us all asks for safety; but instead of heeding the inner pain and calls for help we turn away and continue to self-parent without listening or being present.

As adults it is our responsibility to care for ourselves in a more loving way and support that part of us that requires nurturing. We must say to ourselves,

'I will never again make you feel scared or alone, I will do everything in my power to protect you.'

Making that vow to your inner child is a transforming and alchemical statement. It will move you from a life of poverty to a life of love. You are counting yourself as someone who deserves ultimate peace, security and happiness.

Living with weak protection invites people into your life who allow you to replay old patterns that need healing. We find ourselves in repeated contact with people who drain our energy from us, use us, manipulate us or take us for a ride. We need to learn to toughen up our boundaries and realize we have a right to retain our own power for ourselves. In the absence of real protection we may try and create false boundaries with body weight, dowdy appearance or habitual behaviour patterns. We would rather stay in the background than have people take notice. As we work with protection we create distance from harm and it is easier for us to come out of our shells and liven up. We harness our power and as our confidence grows we move closer towards our own personal truth. In our power, weaker energies will prove no contest. We are free to reserve all our energy for own life purposes.

Working with Protection

Answer these questions honestly:

~ Do I feel safe?
~ If not, why not? What scares me? Who makes me feel unsafe?
~ How confident do I feel when faced with difficult situations?
~ How protected did I feel as a child?

~   Has anything significant happened in my past that may have
    left me with lasting traumatic memories?
~   Do I feel grounded?
~   Do I feel confident to stand out in a crowd or do I try to
    deflect attention from myself?
~   Do I suffer from anxieties, phobias or obsessive thought
    patterns?
~   Am I assertive and independent in relationships?
~   Do I have any self-destructive behaviours that make me feel
    unsafe?

Your answers may highlight trigger points or issues that need
resolving or healing. You may now be aware that you have
certain behaviours or patterns that reflect a level of low
protection.

It is now that you can start the process of change; today is a
new beginning.

Addressing Pain and Trauma

As you become more insightful to areas of pain or disharmony,
you may finally be brave enough to want to change. This takes
courage, patience and dedication and quite often is an all-
consuming and unsettling process. I always advise contacting a
specialized therapist to guide you through the darkness and to
provide support and expertise to facilitate release of pain in the
energy body.

Counsellors, doctors, psychotherapists, homeopaths, healers
and other complementary therapists are all conduits of healing
energy, and once you are committed to your path, forces will
come to your aid to light the way. Have faith and trust your
instincts in choosing the right people to help you at this time.
You must have a certain rapport, as a level of trust, love and
professionalism is vital in those who will be suitably equipped
to empathize with and treat you as you deserve.

The remedies and techniques I work with are all chosen on a
highly individualized basis, and I feel it is always wiser to have

someone objective and sensitive by your side, if you are working to shift deep-buried pain. This is especially relevant where childhood abuse or physical or sexual violation has occurred. It is a deeply emotive area and always one best tackled with a skilled guide. Grieve for the loss or difficulty in your past. Let go of old behaviours. Open to love.

Practising Protection

Positive Intention and Purity of Thought

Purify your own thoughts; cleanse your mind of negativity and anger on a conscious level. Refuse to allow yourself the indulgence of bitterness or blame. Watch for snap judgements on others, critical thinking and thoughts of revenge. Thought forms are felt as subtle energies by others, even though their conscious minds may not process this as fact. Every action has a reaction. By practising self-discipline over the thoughts you have, you protect yourself through the law of karma. You will attract less negativity. Try to detach, don't react – focus on your own path.

Truth, like a fire, will burn through discord and disharmony.

Relinquish thoughts of fear, and believe you are safe and protected

Visualization

Imagine a golden-white light surrounding you like a shield, deflecting negative and harmful energies away from you. Inside, you are safe and quite at peace. When you wake, when you step outside, when you encounter any situation where you need to feel strong, imagine the light around you, protecting you always.

With practice, the density will intensify, you will feel more powerful and the image carried in your mind's eye will stand between you and any outside influence. You may tailor specific layers of your shield to defend against different types of intrusive energy. You can build as many layers as you wish. This is particularly helpful in difficult working situations or relationships where you feel easily influenced. It will enable you to say no, or to stand your ground. After time this will become a sixth sense, you will be amazed that you never thought to protect yourself previously. You should feel your boundaries become more defined and your power increase.

Make a promise to yourself that you will practise this faithfully morning and night for 14 days.

Another important visualization to try is disconnecting and de-cording from others to create integrity in your outer shell. Spend five minutes alone with your thoughts. Close your eyes. If you can, imagine yourself sitting in a stone circle with your golden-white shield surrounding you. Scan the border for any holes, tears or cords. Ask for guidance to release any cords, and cut them carefully, mending any tears with silver light. You may see faces as the cords are cut by the silver light. Send love from your heart, say goodbye and set them free. Severing this connection does not end a relationship but allows healthy detachment and space to move freely. If it is hard to visualize this, don't worry. You can just as easily shut your eyes and ask that this may happen, that you are willing for the changes to take place. Lie at peace until you feel this is complete.

~ Ask for your spirit guides to be with you at all times.
~ Follow your instincts.

Remedy Store

~ Walnut, a Bach's Flower Essence, is very good for cutting ties, increasing protection and reducing the influence of others as you go through transition. Take a few drops morning and evening, until your own protection builds.

~ Black tourmaline, when carried on the person, helps to deflect negative energy. Remember to clean it with fresh water, dry carefully and charge with the intent to protect you personally, before wearing.

~   Black obsidian is also a grounding crystal that strengthens
    our connection to mother earth and our base chakra. It
    allows us to release shadow energy, and enhances
    protection.
~   Electro - an Australian bush flower essence that shields us
    from negative energies, heals damage to our aura and
    increases personal power.

Making Changes

Improve your level of self-care and seek to minimize self-
destructive behaviours at this time. These reflect a weakened
level of protection. Ask yourself why you may want to take
actions that negate your self-worth or cause you poor health or
pain. If you feel the answers lie too deep, seek professional help
to uncover the root cause of your patterns. Examine your
relationships and see if you can identify the healthy and loving
ones. Spend time with those who truly support you and make
you feel safe.

It may help to keep a journal as you work with this and every
Principle, to chart your growth and keep track of your changing
emotions, perceptions and insights.

Global Protection

By increasing our personal protection as individuals we elevate
our Principle globally from one of fear and insecurity to one of
goodwill, grounding and compassion. We become a less hostile
humanity, more trusting, less ready to attack at the slightest
provocation. We think before we act. By practising everyday
protection we raise the universal vibration. Choose love over
fear. Meditate on peace.

Living a Protected Life

Watch for remarkable transformation in your life as you grow in
strength and power and begin to feel freer. To feel truly protected
is to feel nurtured, secure and loved. We learn to fly. It is a call
to honesty about who we really are.

If we are not ready to accept total truth, we are not ready to face our destiny.

We may welcome lower levels of protection to detract from our true path and introduce unhealthy or imbalanced relationships, and to maintain a sense of false closeness and support. We crave something or someone to fill the emptiness for us. We are too scared to stand alone; we are too weak to take responsibility.

Healthy support comes from an actualised individual who has learnt to stand alone; he proves to be a tower of strength, but is no more a drain on your energy than you are on his. He will be compassionate but separate – the difference between co-dependency and true friendship.

As you begin to work with protection you will change internally; it will become apparent to you who your true friends are and this shift requires courage as you reassess who is actually right for you, and ultimately how certain relationships in your past have reflected on yourself.

Be prepared to value yourself and seek independence. You are strong enough.

We are often self-destructive when we fear our own brightness; we are less self-destructive if we reveal our darkness.

What we try and destroy is the human pain we all carry at times, but also the greatness that lives by its side. Don't be afraid of your light, your creativity, your divinity – exalt your gifts and grace.

As your protection grows in definition you will become more defined as a person. There is a clear demarcation between your spiritual essence and that of the world. You shine in your uniqueness, proud to be different. You no longer need validation from others, or the external trappings of fitting in. You are confident, comfortable and entirely present. It becomes less about what others think and more about you. You are governed by your own principles and right action.

Protection

~ Protection is the First Principle of Light.

~ Protection is intrinsic to the strength and development of our energy system.

~ Protection builds and concentrates character and spiritual essence.

~ Protection is necessary to shield us from negativity and harm.

~ Protection allows us to express ourselves in our total truth.

~ Protection breeds power, healthy relationships, creativity and grounding.

~ Protection enables us to move towards our soul destiny.

~ Protection maintains the security of the inner child.

~ Protection is magnified with purity of thought and right action.

~ Protection that is weakened attracts negative situations or people that may drain us or harm us.

~ Protection is a reflection of our self-esteem and how much we consider ourselves worthy of safety.

~ Protection promotes detachment and compassion.

~ Protection is your home.

~ Protection is divine introspection.

~ Protection calls for living within.

~ Protection is the crowning leaves that cradle the bloom.

~ The golden cup that holds the nectar.

~ The holy spark in the moving fire.

~ The unborn child in a mother's womb.

~ Value yourself every day.

~ You are infinitely precious.

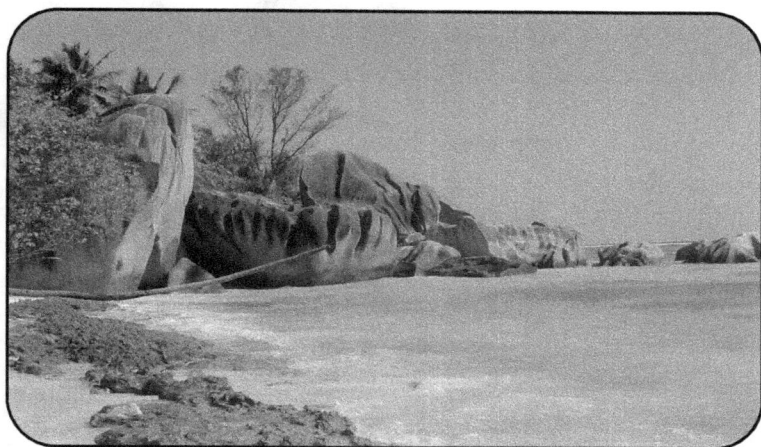

2

Abundance

Abundance is the second Principle of Light. Abundance is the garden that grows within the walls of your protection, your paradise kingdom whence the well of vitality and life springs. In individual terms it is the essence of what your soul requires and desires for growth and harmony.

In a dreamscape, abundance may appear as lush wilderness, rolling green hills and pastures, bright colours, blue skies, man, animal and environment unified. It is Gaia created as vibrant world energy, existing in perfect synchronicity. Abundance is akin to fertility, prosperity, joy, and our cups brimming over. We have enough of what we need and what we need will flow to us like a river to the sea. We are willing to share in our wellbeing because as we give so shall we receive.

Our life force carries us from destination to destination and as we trust in the energy that gives us existence so we trust that

same energy to bring us peace, health and wealth. We have faith
in abundance that the universe will deliver unto us our destiny.

Why Abundance is Important

Abundance represents the torch of survival as the human race
continues to populate the planet. Abundance represents all things
which support us in our growth; money, food, shelter and love.
It also has a direct relation to our vital force, our life spark, our
very will that pushes us to survive against all the odds. It
governs how confident we are in supporting ourselves and
standing on our own two feet. How strong do we feel when both
our feet are on the ground; are we shaky or do we stand poised
and graceful? Does the universal energy coursing from the earth
up and through us as spirit, connect with us as one?

When we access abundance energy, and all the world has to
offer, we fire on all cylinders, our engine propels us on our life
path as slowly or quickly as we choose. There is never any
question that we are too tired, can't be bothered, don't care. That
very energy makes us alert, inquisitive, responsive and proactive
in our quest, it sails us down the river. We explore, experience
and discover a life that makes us excited and happy, and use this
energy to build a space around us that harmonizes with our inner
truth.

For many, abundance is symbolized purely in material terms.
To me, abundance is far more than just the trappings of wealth.
An abundant life is one where love is intertwined with all its
facets. Money is a part of the picture and readily facilitates
freedom and growth, but if those experiences are not directed
with heart energy, to the end creation of a heaven where the soul
sings, you may find yourself living an incomplete existence,
yearning for the missing piece in an apparently perfect life.

Love is always first, love for yourself and the gifts you can
bring to your heart, and love for others with the joy, warmth and
blessings that enrich you through sharing relationships. There is
a responsibility that comes with true abundance, a karma that
runs deep in all the Principles; growth must be fostered in

accordance with others and the earth energy. It cannot occur at the expense of others' misfortune as this detracts from the principle of abundant flow.

May we all move together towards a higher state of harmony.

To understand abundance is to walk a wiser path, to open your eyes and senses to the flow of the life cycle and the unending spiritual meaning in all things, however stark or materialistic they may seem. Move your focus from finite terms to a generous and nurturing universe that wants you to prosper. Believe in that and believe in your happiness.

Ask your soul now. What does it truly sing for?

How does Abundance Develop?

Abundance as a Principle is a mirror of our very early experiences and karma as we enter the planet as an incarnated soul. As old souls, we may have memories laid down in our karmic bonds of very different life experiences, but our conscious recollections will be based on the imprint of our early life. The energy that we carry through from one lifetime to the next is relevant to our current incarnation; it will dictate our well of experiences to draw knowledge from, and the strength and nature of our divine spark.

Our vitality is reflected in our general health and constitution and our ability to weather physical, emotional and spiritual challenges; in other words, our ability to endure. It is easy to see vitality when you look for it; the divine spark shining from the eyes, a glow or radiance from the skin that issues from within, a genuine love of humanity and existence. Children have this light and will continue to burn with this fire as long as they stay close to their purpose and remain on their path in their road to adulthood.

We often give up our search for abundance as the heavy burden of sorrow or pain becomes weighted in our field, and until we transform this to the higher energies of love the view can be very cloudy; we forget the green fields and rainbows of our youthful wishes. We may forget that we deserve to experience the best and lose our way, creating and maintaining a semblance of deprivation in our life as a mirror of what we believe we are worth in our unhappy state.

We may also choose to squander our natural energy, allowing it to become scattered and unfocussed. We do this without realizing that without fire in our loins we find it hard to harness and direct our will effectively. When we are healthy, emotionally and physically, our life force makes us want to get up and go, leap with excitement, run, dance, work and play. We have passion. This energy is universal and fundamental – we all share the same stream.

How we manifest abundance mirrors our life energy and our early conditioning. These environmental factors and messages play a big part during childhood and young adulthood in how we view the world picture and our place on that map. If we were born into money and comfort, subconsciously we may assume that the world is a safe place where it is easy to obtain what we need. On the other hand, if times were hard and it was difficult to get by or put food on the table, it is understandable that we may grow to doubt our ability to survive in a world where circumstances are unpredictable. The beliefs of our parents may also play a part; how comfortable they felt in managing financial or material energy would imprint to some degree on how much you fear or trust the universe to provide a safe and abundant haven. Did they give and receive easily? Were they frightened of the power of money? Did they use it to manipulate you or gain control? Did they push it away or fritter it because they did not feel they deserved the riches in life? Did you feel it would be wrong to leave certain expectations or limitations behind for fear of outgrowing your family, or did you push away the value of abundance because you felt the way it was portrayed in your upbringing was a negative thing?

Finding your own way and your own essence is important. Elevating the Principle of abundance through love is the only way to achieve true balance, where monetary gain is only a part of what abundance really means to you. Abundance is all about having what you choose, and what you dream of in accordance with the grand design. What would truly make you happy is a set of deeply held experiences that equal a blissful earthly existence, not a big pile of money. Money can make things happen, but many of life's pleasures are instead created from having more time, more love, and more freedom. With self-development, other people's ideas and fears drop away and what you are left with is self-knowledge; how you would like to use your power.

It is absolutely necessary to discard that which does not support you. It is imperative you continue to dream and desire. Those inner wishes are expressions and facets of your individuality and as you manage to grow, from correct use of your vital energy, your expression of life will grow increasingly abundant. Don't be afraid of your mighty energy; try not to dissipate your reserves. Instead use it to water the dormant seeds that lie within. What starts as a bud, if nurtured correctly, will bloom into the most beautiful and fragrant flower if you believe in yourself.

~ Recognize your vitality, life force, drive and inner will.
~ Remain grounded and supported by the earth's energy.
~ Realize the force of your fire.
~ Fan the flame to create warmth and energy.
~ Direct the flame to achieve direction.
~ Transform your spiritual fire into your dreams.
~ Live on earth as if you are living in heaven.

With such positive expectation and exploration, opportunities arise from nowhere. We thrive.

When Abundance is Strong

When abundance is strong, we have a sense of completeness, richness and joy in our lives. We look around and feel security, warmth and love. We are cradled in the supportive arms of Mother Earth and all that she provides. We have no doubt that what we need to foster growth will be given, that indeed as we progress through life growth will occur effortlessly, as naturally as the acorn becomes the oak. We have enough.

We understand the nature of money as purely an energy flow. We have no fear or judgement regarding what it represents but use it to provide nourishment and freedom as that energy is transmuted into another form of life.

So we grow by granting ourselves the necessary experiences from which to learn as we travel, and ground ourselves as we journey by developing sufficient stability and support. We put our roots down so we may feel secure as we mature. As we branch out into new territory we know we will not topple or fall. There is no sense of negative or positive when we look at money objectively. What is negative or positive is how we use it and what we seek to gain from it.

We are able to give and receive in equal measure in tune with the law of karma.

We support ourselves first and then we reach out to help a brother in need. We understand that by giving unconditionally, the universe will return, and abundance energy will flow back to us, as we require aid and assistance.

We do not fear the power of prosperity. We are stronger than it and are wise and respectful when handling our affairs. We trust ourselves to make the right choices in alignment with right action. We spend and save without hoarding or frittering.

Our hands hold gently and give easily.

We are brave enough to enjoy the energy of abundance without it overpowering us. We revel in the adventures it affords us and are generous with others.

Our paradise is a haven within our garden walls, an oasis watered with our vital spirit, a place of harmony and happiness where we are present in our incarnation.

We use our resources with intelligence and dignity and have the utmost respect for the world at large.

We support others as we support ourselves, and in turn, our universe supports us all.

When Abundance is Weak

We exist in poverty consciousness.

The world fails to provide for us, it takes from us; there is never enough. We fear daily for our survival, our safety, our lives.

We feel disempowered in our ability to create prosperity. We disassociate the energy of abundance from ourselves and it becomes a separate, frightening, uncontrollable force, greater than ourselves. We cannot win. We maintain low expectations and feel we deserve little from life, setting our internal mental comfort zone at a level that we think befits our worth. We may carry imprinted beliefs that equate to our present circumstances, someone else's standards of what life has to offer, or what is reasonable to hope for.

Money becomes anti-spiritual, the root of all evil, something dark that leads to difficulty and destruction. We fail to distance the neutrality of abundance energy from the judgements projected by man's shadow. We push prosperity away, turn our back on opportunities and engender situations or relationships that drain our abundance energy from us. There is a balance in giving and receiving – to give is good but when we give at the expense of our own vitality the exchange is based on fear and not love, as we are denying our own existence and needs.

Maybe we feel money is the only answer to all our problems and seek to gain material riches beyond all else; the pursuit of wealth negating the value of relationships, love or self-knowledge. Financial accumulation becomes a holy grail. It is used as a negative energy; to manipulate, gain authority and keep others in a position of subservience. Relationships are based on a transaction: control for apparent security. Both have entered into a low energy bond as the vibration fails to create heart energy. The ties that bind come at a price, as without the expression of unconditional love, the fire of abundance is extinguished – the semblance of happiness is there without the true warmth at the centre. One person buys; the other allows himself to be bought.

Money is used unethically; theft, criminal activity, arms dealing, slavery, political subterfuge, the list is endless. Again material energy is exchanged at a low vibrational plane, creating discord and misery; a few benefit from the denial of many.

We have a responsibility in how we use our money, individually and as a nation. What does it create? Where does it go? Where does our abundance energy flow – to create growth or to deplete humanity? Ask yourself this – are we being just?

The nature of giving and receiving is poorly grasped. The amassment of money solely for power becomes gospel in our society, greed with no actual end.

We are all entitled to earn and create and provide but if that aim is purely to attain power over others, then this core belief is again at odds with abundance energy.

Money can equal power, but only prosperity and love equal abundance. In that love we consider others and we grow with love. We are not separate from the others in our world, we are not trying to compete to boost a fragile ego. We do not have to prove we are lovable by having to be better and greater than everyone else; we can just be. We are unique and strong in our individuality. In a humane society we hope to prosper and attain our dreams and wishes but part of those dreams is to exist in a society where everyone has a chance in life, of happiness and health, where our growth does not come at the expense of others.

By believing in greed, we believe in finite resources – we need to hold on to everything we have for fear of not having enough, or of what we have being taken from us. The more we have the safer we will be. This way of thinking excludes the right for everyone to have enough – prosperity becomes a privilege instead of a human right. It does not detract from the democratic right to run a business or become successful through productivity; what it means is that we should consider the nature of our economic growth and use our fortune to benefit our community and our world – industry reflected as an ethical statement.

The other side of the coin is that many push abundance away by confusing it with the notion of greed. They fear the power of wealth and freedom and the effect it may have on their lives, and they don't want the responsibility that comes with power. As long as prosperity is coupled with conscience it becomes a positive force for good and growth, as with higher intentions this energy can be utilized to manifest necessary planetary expansion and progression. Those who feel they are unworthy or frightened of abundance may drain it away by gambling, overspending or poor management. They feel the happiness and stability created by material stability is beyond them.

World View

One question that remains unanswered is the subject of world poverty. Millions are born into harsh and hostile circumstances where fighting for survival is a reality and no amount of wishing will change their path. These incarnated souls do not have the choice of building abundance – theirs is a fate of hunger, despair and fear on a daily basis.

I can only explain the truth behind this complex situation as I see it, which you may choose to disagree with. I believe that souls living in poverty carry our world shadow. They are a mirror of the poverty consciousness that exists in the richer nations – they are a fundamental opposite to the greedy thinking in the West that denies equality in abundance. People living in both circumstances believe there isn't enough, both believe in finite resources. One man will hang on to what he can, and as much as he can, the other goes without. There is no sharing, no growth with love, no economic responsibility, no awareness of anything but the self.

In recent times we have started to become more aware of the imbalance that exists, and that cannot exist in our world conscience any longer. We are a humane society and we therefore ask for an end to demands from the already rich for continuing debt repayment from impoverished populations. We are unhappy about what governments choose to spend our money on; the distribution of budgets appears unethical and misguided. We now take responsibility as educated citizens to send aid to the suffering overseas as one disaster after another wipes out entire communities or generations. We watch news footage of these political and natural devastations and the message is brought home; we must do what we can. We can no longer sit by and pretend a lack of connection, we care and we care deeply. We are ready to stop the fighting; we want to heal.

We may not be able to change the cultural and political fabric of foreign countries at all, we may be frustrated by the structures that continue to bring misfortune to so many. We cannot begin to understand the way another man's reality truly is. But we can try. We can keep our hearts open and keep trying.

If we have the privilege to be born into an abundant society it is also our responsibility to use that abundance wisely. Karma is coming round. In this new era there has already been dramatic change; the New Age demands a shift from poverty consciousness to one of universal connection and compassion.

Every child in this universe deserves shelter, food, education, medicine, sanitation, warmth and love.

What are we doing to make this happen?

Open the door to global abundance – spread the wealth.

Working with Abundance

Answer these questions honestly:

~ How abundant is my life? How is my garden growing?
~ Do I have enough? If not, what is missing? How could I change this?
~ What are my intrinsic beliefs about money?
~ What did I learn about abundance and money when I was growing up?
~ Do I feel I can support myself? Do I allow others to support me? Does the universe support me?
~ Do I have enough energy?

~ Do I ever feel manipulated by money? Do I allow myself to be bought?
~ What symbolizes abundant living to me? (Be specific and ask yourself what you really would like in your landscape.)
~ How can I go about achieving my dream?
~ Am I responsible with money, can I handle it or am I afraid?
~ Do I find it easy to give and easy to receive in equal measure?

If you find one area or both difficult, ask yourself why this is.

Think carefully about your responses and notice certain patterns and imprinting within your belief system. Remember your thoughts create the universe, influence the choices you make and the opportunities you take, and are a measure of what you feel you deserve. It is time to wash away those beliefs that do not belong to you, do not support you and stand in the way of your ideal of abundance. If you feel energies begin to shift internally, let them rise. Notice anger and/or pain as they surface and observe quietly. It may help to write them down as they appear; insight fosters acceptance and separation.

It is easy to move on if you truly want to. Discover what stays with you, what you can change, what you can now do to move from point A to point B. Map it in your mind step by step. There is always a way, always a higher path if you dare to dream.

Believe in the abundance you deserve.

You are infinitely more powerful than you could imagine.

Practising Abundance

Harnessing Natural Energy Flow
Sit cross-legged on the ground on a blanket, sit on a chair or stand. Imagine earth energy entering from the ground up through the soles of your feet to your legs, up to the base of the spine, or if you are sitting, straight to the base of the spine. Let it collect at the root and flow upward, up the spine, right to the crown of

your head. As it reaches the top let it run back down the spine as you repeat the action in circular motion. You might want to close your eyes as you do this and visualize the energy as a golden or silver light. Each time you reach the base of the spine see yourself picking up a little more earth energy as you continue. Imagine this to be universal abundance energy and practise feeling that connection between yourself and the planet.

Feel yourself becoming more and more energized. How much energy can you gather? This is an energy which is yours to harness, run, let it course through you. Feel its power, feel your power. Let it circle through your system, up your spine and down, and back again. How much abundance energy can you carry? Be aware of any blocks or discomfort in any particular region of flow. These areas may indicate that a chakra needs clearing of stagnant energy. Any energetic congestion may prevent you from accepting powerful universal force. Let yourself flow for as long as you want and remember to hold that energy within you when you finish.

Self-Care

Improve your nutrition and exercise plan. Eat wisely and breathe deeply. Regular exercise builds strength and rids your body of toxins. It builds warrior energy. Health promotes vitality and a natural sense of confidence and abundance. Pump up the volume of your personal energy and maximize your life potential. Have some respect for your body, as your energy is now your wealth.

Manifestation

Draw your abundance paradise on paper or in your mind's eye. Write down the key things that would make your world an abundant one. Remember to keep your expectations individual and personal.

What do you see in your future dream? See it clearly. It may represent different things – money yes, but more importantly what that represents to you. A new home, time off from work, travel, children, new experiences and freedom. Write trigger words and draw symbols. Be creative and don't be too afraid to dream.

Each time you drift into poverty thinking, remember your dream. Channel your energy into power thinking instead of letting it translate to fear. Get into the flow of abundance energy; trust the world to guide you. Start making small plans to take you where you would like to go. Ask the universe to guide you. Be willing to ask for what you dream of; being afraid to ask for fear of not receiving sends out negative signals, blocking your dreams from manifestation.

Affirmations

Write a long list of the negative messages you carry regarding your right to abundance or money on one half of a piece of paper. When you have done this, by the side of each one write a positive message to replace it. For example, you could replace 'money is a dangerous thing' with 'money is a positive thing which helps me to grow'. Do this for each one. When you have finished, tear the page in half and destroy the negative messages. Either rip them up or burn them in a safe way or simply throw them away with intention. You are making the way for new supportive ways of thinking.

Ask the universe to aid clearance from your energy system. Carry the positive ones with you for the next week. Let them sink into your subconscious. Read them twice a day. Allow them to become your new reality. However unrealistic this seems at the time, try not to judge yourself. Keep up the practice. If you feel a negative message floating up, observe it and let it go. Repeat a positive statement in your mind straight away.

Keep repeating your positive messages on a regular basis. Keep believing.

Giving and Receiving

Practise giving to charity – even if it is only a small amount, giving a little to a good cause engenders a sense of positive karma and builds your trust in abundance energy. Do this on a regular basis and the universe will reward you. Give what you can afford and give with grace and good intent.

Remedy Store

Flower essences
~   Abund essence (combination Australian Bush Flower) enhances belief in abundance.

Crystals
~   Citrine is a warm, yellow amber crystal, which encourages vitality and abundance.
~   The colour red is invigorating to the root chakra, so wearing ruby or other red stones strengthens this centre.

Oils
~   Cinnamon oil warms the root chakra.

~   Laughing Buddha - not so much a remedy, but an artefact often found in new age shops. I find that mine has definitely brought me prosperity in all parts of life.

Living an Abundant Life
Abundance is a state of mind.

As you move from a narrow worldview to one of openness and sweetness, everything changes. The world is simply your oyster; anything becomes possible. Once you access the vital energy that is open to us all, you will encounter a drive and a spark that gets you up each morning, ready to greet a brand new day with excitement and hope. You will begin to feel your childlike wonder and excitement return.

Working through old values and limitations takes courage and dedication but therein lays the power to align your existence with your inner potential. It can be hard to let go of the beliefs which you feel may protect you from disappointment or failure: 'If I don't want too much, I won't be upset when it doesn't happen'. But if you choose to live a life in fear you prevent all chance of attaining what is rightfully yours. Reach out and touch your dreams. Taste the possibility. Adventure!

The flow of abundance will begin to carry you on your journey – the flow meanders within the confines of realistic possibility but brings sparkle and excitement with benefits and blessings appearing from nowhere. You will start to travel the Warrior's way; your life will become colourful and richer in the very depth and fabric of your day-to-day ways.

You will become more aware that there is a source that continues to provide, a pot that doesn't run out, as you begin to respect the Principle of abundance and work with it instead of pushing it away or acting from a place of fear. There is intrinsic synchronicity. There are natural tides, what goes out comes in and as you give so you shall receive.

Abundance relates to freehearted generosity and giving. It excludes manipulation, money used for harm or unethical gain. Karma will balance that which takes away – there is a freedom in being honest and righteous as you grow with this Principle. You may make mistakes along the way but forgive yourself as the universe will forgive you and make a fresh start each day.

When you understand what true abundance is for you as an individual being it will be easier and less complicated to travel light. Take only what you need to grow and things will become simple.

Prosperity is golden and with it you may achieve material stability from where it is truly possible to embrace the mission of your soul incarnation. When we are aligned in our motives the energy is there to come together and push our universe through to the next dimension, where abundance and harmony reign throughout. Imagine the joy we could bring, the paradise we could create.

Pray each day for abundance – clear your own negative messages and begin to believe with openness and wonder.

Abundance

~ Abundance is the second Principle of Light.

~ Abundance is an expression of life, which befits your individual spiritual nature.

~ Abundance is always intertwined with love.

~ Abundance is linked to the root chakra and is integral to our personal vitality and power.

~ Abundance is a flow of energy, which, in health, fosters growth and trust in the universal supply.

~ Abundance becomes poverty consciousness in its negative expression.

~ Abundance is directly related to the law of giving and receiving.

~ We have a responsibility to use our power and money wisely and respectfully.

~ Abundance reflects our internal self-esteem and what we feel we deserve from life.

~ Abundance when separated from love becomes purely material. Man's shadow projections lower the vibration to diminished fear-based energy.

~ Abundance beliefs are often imprinted in childhood and relate to how well we were nurtured and supported.

We have a global responsibility to push our universe from poverty consciousness to a reign of abundance.

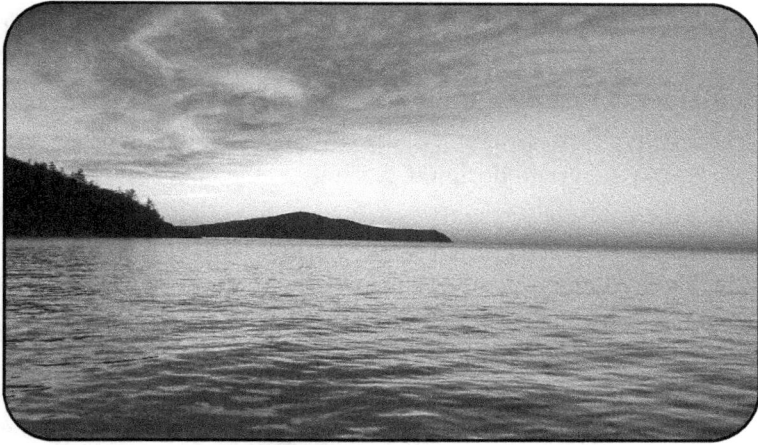

3

Creativity

Welcome Creativity as the Third Principle of Light. Creativity brings lightening, laughter, magic and sweetness to our life energy. With creative energy we discover we were born to have fun. Creativity shakes up our natural vitality into a colourful display of divine self-expression. We discover and delight in our gifts and talents as they draw us to our divinity. We marvel in the beauty and wonder of our uniqueness. This is abundance energy channelled into play, passion, adventure and happiness, everything that makes us tick, gets us going, makes our life worth living.

Creativity shows us what interests us, what fascinates us and what inspires us. By doing this, it shows us ourselves. We all define the masterpiece that depicts the glorious diversity of humanity. Man has an innate compulsion to build, make, invent – to create something from nothing.

Creativity allows us the method to explore the world and find ourselves through our desires – it gives our lives depth, richness and magnificence. We lose ourselves when we fall effortlessly into creative flow. Creativity is essentially spiritual. Creativity is integral to the grand design. Creativity is the dance of life.

Why Creativity is Important

It is the rhythm in our story, the song that plays as a backdrop to our memories, the exhilaration and sheer brilliance of living.

With creativity we build miracles – the thought becomes an idea, becomes a plan and becomes a reality. A seed grows to a bud, to a shoot and then to a flower. It is the cycle of life – creation. It is as intrinsic to our human state as the creation of our earth, the development of our civilization, the onward and upward expansion and growth inherent to mankind. This power drives us forward in ever-increasing possibilities – with each new soul incarnating to our universe come fresh ideas and ways of thinking, with each generation come new ways of being and doing, living and seeing. We have come a long way, because we all have this desire to create as part of our being. To be is to do and to do is to create.

We are powerful people with a strong urge to bring forth from ourselves, be it through cooking, painting, writing, dancing, designing, singing ... the list is endless. These are activities that are often less about work but more about who we are and what we enjoy doing. In our pastimes, in alignment with our creative urge, we lose ourselves, we are free. We create because we can, because we must, because we are. We were born to enjoy the journey of life and travel into the light with peace and laughter, to play and experience, to have fun with each other as we learn along the way. We are all able to exude a sense of wonder in the power of others as well as to acknowledge and respect the outstanding presence we carry within. To nurture and develop our own gifts is to recognize our creativity as the divine within all of us – an alchemical magic from which we are all able to reproduce new life in whatever shape or form comes naturally to us.

The mastery of creative energy by man gives birth to everything we need to develop further as a unified civilization as well as providing a splash of vibrancy and splendour to proceedings.

Creativity beholds the art in life.

How does Creativity Develop?

Creativity is never more apparent in its pure form than in childhood. Children learn through the art of play and exploration and love all things noisy, messy colourful and active. They are enthralled by light, colour, sound and movement and have an obvious sense of satisfaction and achievement from producing and building different things. They enjoy the process of creation for creation's sake, not for the end result of being judged on how good it is, but because they truly gained and found pleasure in their chosen activity. They put their own stamp on each piece of 'work', put a healthy dose of themselves into it. They naturally gravitate to what they feel comfortable and happy with but are usually willing to try different things. They go with the flow, ever delighting in the simplicity of play.

Early childhood is a stage of life where the pressures of school reports or ensuing deadlines have not yet made their mark. All creative efforts are praised and judgement is generally absent as part of the creativity equation. At this age, the normal response is to praise everything with awe and amazement, as we are not looking at technical flair, but the brilliance in the translation of thought into art. We are praising the creative process.

As we get older our efforts are generally met with a more critical eye. We also begin our rocky passage through adolescence into adulthood. As we travel the road to maturity there may be plentiful opportunities to suffer at the hand of an unkind word or harsh opinion from someone who is usually mirroring his own blocked creativity or self-esteem. If self-

esteem is shattered at a young age it can have a lasting impact
on how valuable we feel ourselves to be, how worthy our best
efforts are, how valid our actions and opinions are and how able
we feel to stand out in a crowd and be counted. We learn to feel
shame.

Shame is the antithesis to self-esteem. Shame is the moment
when we feel less than the truly wondrous child of the universe
we are. A child raised with enough unconditional love and
support will brush off critics and start again, but a child who has
become ashamed of who they are will be frightened to hold their
heads high, and will not feel equal. The creative urge is primal,
but if the basic self-confidence is not there to support it a child
may grow into an adult who is too afraid to even try, suppressing
any natural ability for fear of exposing their core inadequacy.
Some souls are born with prodigal gifts and against the odds
they do achieve creatively, but the taint of shame may express
itself in other areas of their lives; an inability to manage their
talent without self-destructing or a deeper unhappiness despite
external appearances of success.

So creativity and self-esteem are linked in development.
Together great things follow.

We all experience some degree of shame in our lives but the
road to light asks you to clear any negativity you feel about
yourself, any difficulty you may have in accepting yourself, and
any pain you feel from allowing others to see the beautiful
person you really are inside.

We forget our creative nature with age, pretend we never had
it or it wasn't ours to keep. We deny the energy we all possess
that takes pride and happiness in expanding our skills, learning
and developing through every age. Work becomes our focus and
too often work is a mechanical, repetitive logical affair that
necessitates our existence.

Our soul sings for more but maybe all we need to do is find
that rhythm again, the simple joy of realizing our power to bring
magic into the world. To create for creation's sake, in any way,

shape or form we choose, without self-doubt, self-criticism or fear of judgement.

~ Creativity shines with a glorious golden orange glow.
~ Creativity lives in Swadistana, the Home of the Self.
~ We worship the god and the goddess within.
~ We are radiant with love, we are vibrant with pleasure.
~ We are comfortable in our own skin.
~ We know passion for life.
~ We know happiness, joy, laughter and light.
~ Life is for living, my friend.
~ Life is for having fun.
~ Life is magical.

When Creativity is Strong

~ We are exuberant, alive and ecstatic.
~ We smile and laugh and understand the humour in everyday experience.
~ We have a lust for life, a passion for what excites us and we live and breathe to be involved, to be active, to watch things grow from our own making.
~ We love colour and diversity, new tastes, sights and sounds.
~ We are in tune with our senses but we retain a position of mastery over them.
~ We are directed and focussed with our creativity; we can concentrate and channel the fountain of life to transform natural creative energy into a reflection of our essence.
~ What we create is a picture of what we already hold within formed with divine universal flow.
~ We create with beauty.
~ We are beauty – we acknowledge the beauty in ourselves as one of life's greatest creations – humankind.
~ We have esteem for ourselves, our health, our abilities – we look upon ourselves with love.
~ We feel connected and empowered in our sexuality, our physical bodies and our current incarnation.

~   We appreciate the magnitude of our personal power and nurture it, using it wisely – we do not fear it or deplete it but treat it with the utmost respect, as a gift from God. With this power we continue to create ourselves.

~   We strive to transform negative thinking and self-defeating patterns and grow to live with confidence and courage.

~   We are gentle with ourselves, encouraging our own creative efforts as if we were still that small child painting a picture for the first time.

~   We cast no judgement on others' attempts in self-expression.

~   We replace shame with pride in what we can do and who we were born to be.

~   We are vibrant, colourful, ripe and fertile with possibility and potential.

~   We are comfortable with our perceived imperfections as they are what make us unique.

~   We are each a small part of the bigger picture and we are all loved in the eyes of the universe.

When Creativity is Weak

Our creative force is imbalanced or diminished.

We may have suffered early traumatic experiences that hindered our ability to develop in harmony with our creative wellspring.

Our self-esteem is low and we feel disconnected from our physical bodies, at odds with the power that resides within us. We may turn from it, suppress it, diminish it or fear it.

Our society supports us in this defeatist behaviour by promoting cosmetic surgery, crash dieting and the beauty industry. The inner dissatisfaction in the soul becomes projected onto the shell.

We think that by becoming more externally attractive we become more lovable, will gain more love, will lose the shame we feel and become more worthy. By changing our outward appearance we may gain societal recognition, but unless the soul needs are addressed, we will not receive the unconditional love from others or ourselves, which is how we truly find peace.

There is a difference between healthy self-respect and self-care, delighting in our individuality, beauty and sexuality and a belief system that is based on insecurity, and the underlying supposition that you are not good enough the way you are. This is a sentiment that is rooted in shame.

If we gave as much effort and attention to caring for our inner worlds and needs, the rewards that would be gained would be truly phenomenal. Strip away the inner darkness and what you will find is a deep and abiding love that conquers any semblance of inadequacy.

Love is greater than fear and always will be.

We may develop self-destructive tendencies or hide away from life.

We may exist in a purely rational mindset, separated from our intrinsic creative nature, our ability to bring forth from ourselves feats of wonder and magnificence.

We find ways of expressing our discomfort with ourselves, our shame with who we are.

We run from our demons rather than confront them.

Nothing is ever solved by putting a lid on it.

We may travel on our journey into light experiencing both extremes of unbalanced creativity. We may vault from hedonistic excess to periods of abstinence and self-control.

Creativity flows in the middle path; it is not an effort to exist but a joy to be.

Our passions change with the seasons of our lives; if they are right for us at that time, they bring us closer to our purpose and ourselves. That which takes away, destroys or weakens our force is without spirit or love.

We must appreciate our own life cycle, what is right and correct for us in each moment – we must be honest about our motives and at all times have a handle on what we need to support us now. We grow and change and, as we mature, we will need every ounce of our creative force to burn brightly.

A passion based on fear or pain is an addiction.

Addictions are a metaphor for running away from pain – something else becomes a focal occupation that diverts and drains energy away from confronting the actual truth. The addiction becomes a crutch at first, something to distract from an inner restlessness, dissatisfaction or unhappiness, but soon creates a multitude of problems of its own making. At the heart of each addiction lies a feeling of fear and worthlessness and often a deeply buried pain that its owner is too scared to confront. The longer it is left, however, the more feelings of inadequacy and poverty mount; as an addiction takes root the fabric of life takes on a darker tone and it becomes harder and harder to separate the ugliness of the addictive behaviour from the struggling soul inside.

Addictions ask you to take responsibility and realize your self-worth. Often the most creative people are those that struggle with addictive behaviour. The power at their disposal is immense and sometimes just too much to cope with wisely, as their inner sense of self-worth falters.

We all struggle with some addictive behaviour from time to time.

We become separate from our natural creative urge quite early in life; the shame we all learn to experience is all too easy to hide under layers of personality. We forget how to just be, to expect others to accept us exactly as we are because we accept ourselves. We stop seeing ourselves as immensely creative beings and identify our passions purely with our sexual nature or pleasure-seeking behaviour. This limits the scope of personal potential quite markedly as there is so much more to each of us when we strip away our learned and societal behaviours and move closer to our spiritual or creative selves. Then creativity becomes a unified force, and masculine and feminine energies are inherently balanced in each of us no matter which incarnation we have taken in this lifetime. We have multiple strengths and many gifts. We are self-creative rather than self-destructive and find it easy to achieve harmony between productivity and pleasure.

Sexuality, Kundalini, spiritual fire and creative energy; these are all sparks of the same universal energy that drives our very existence. Embrace and glory in the life force that exists within you.

What we often fear is not the limited value of our existence but the intense and amazing potential we all carry. We are afraid that it is too great for us, we cannot handle it, live up to its potential day after day; we fear we are not enough. We must trust that to each of us a gift is given for the sole purpose of our enjoyment and pleasure. We were all born with something special.

Sexual Trauma

I have chosen to mention this topic separately because of the complexity of the subject matter and the effect it has on the energy body, self-esteem and emotional development. It encompasses a realm of experience from the smallest incident to years of repeated transgression. It affects the very young and the very old, both male and female, and is still handled in our society with a range of emotional responses from denial and disbelief to mass hysteria. It is incredibly common; nearly one in three women are affected in their lives in some way - the numbers less so with men. But despite this staggering frequency it still carries the mantle of a taboo topic and many victims are too frightened or fearful to seek help, trapped with their secret, not knowing which way to turn.

The memory of trauma lives on in the energy body; the victim may for some time have little conscious awareness of the event as the active brain blocks recollection until the person chooses to confront the past. Sometimes the memories will come flooding back in crisis, without warning, and the victim will experience meltdown as the pressure cooker explodes.

The victim may have intense feelings of fear, mistrust, shame, guilt and self-loathing. They may feel cut off from normal society and unable to communicate the tragedy that lives on within, silenced by the horror. They may either exhibit suppression of sexual energy, or sexual needs which partly mirror past experience, as an attempt to relive the trauma through sexual activity. Depending on the parties involved in the assault there may be terror at confronting the truth as this shakes up all previously held beliefs relating to relationships and love; many victims are assaulted by people they know, often when they are too young to seek independence or find an alternative safe haven. The creative power is disconnected and the victim may cope by using addictions or other behaviours to run from the deep-seated pain and confusion. They may develop physical symptoms relating to the sacral region that lead to overactive medical investigation, or seek out unhealthy sexual relationships or interaction, which often result in further damage, and the traumatic cycle deepens.

This is a universal problem.
This is a problem that is still not dealt with wisely.

We vilify the abuser, but we do not deal effectively with the problem on a grand scale. Many abusers were once abused themselves as children, and propagate the cycle by reliving the hand they were dealt. If the cycle is not broken in time, the pain gets handed on; victims may not be driven to inflict harm on others, but at the very least, they experience difficulty with their primary relationships as they struggle to cope with issues of trust, self-worth and intimacy.

We need to accept the problem with maturity as the first and foremost priority should be to make help accessible, to take away the stigma, to allow all victims to step forward and reclaim their dignity. We need to look at the issue from a more adult perspective and help those that need it instead of diverting our energies to persecution of the few. We need to remove shame from the equation, as by doing so we free those who are too scared to open up and tell the truth. It takes courage to embark on the long road to recovery and as a society we need to be ready to listen and accept with wisdom and compassion.

Working with Creativity

The core elements of sacral health are self-esteem, sexuality, creative flow, fun and laughter. It is a glorious, uninhibited, playful energy that we all have the ability to experience as adults. In working with our creative nature, we need to peel away the surrounding layers that we accumulate over time, and revert back to our true essence. This is when we realize our soul gifts and personal life mission and feel peace as we live in our rightful incarnation, without limitation or judgement. From this point of power we will reawaken true passion and excitement for living. Passion will become a far-reaching experience and not one merely limited to our intimate relationships or cravings.

At each point, prepare to let go of unsupportive patterns, own up to the behaviours you use to cope with pain, and let yourself breathe more freely. Let go. Give yourself the unconditional love required to accept yourself deeply, exactly as you are.

Answer these questions honestly:

~ Are you creative?

~ Are you passionate about your life?

~ Do you hold any negative attitudes towards yourself, your abilities, your appearance, your personality?

~ Where do these beliefs originate? Do others imprint them or do you believe them of yourself?

~ Are you prepared to let them go for a new way of thinking? If not, why not?

~ Do you feel comfortable with your appearance and physicality?

~ Do you respect your physical health?

~ If not, could you nurture yourself in any way that increases your level of self-esteem?

~ Are you sexually balanced?

~   Have you ever suffered any sexual trauma? If so, are you
    seeking help or are you ready to start the process?
~   Have you ever been in an unhealthy relationship dynamic
    which affected your self-esteem?
~   Do you have any addictions? What do you think they
    represent?

I recommend that if you do have any issues relating to
addictions, traumatic relationship patterns or sexual abuse, you
should seek specialist help, as you may require psychological
input for some time as you travel the road to recovery. You may
choose a psychoanalyst, a treatment centre, doctors or
counselling services but other therapies may be of use too.
Bodywork, homeopathy, healing and acupuncture are all
valuable in helping to release negative energies from your field.
Choose disciplines that appeal to you and that you feel drawn to.
    I have worked with many patients in the guise of GP,
psychiatrist, homeopath and healer and find the most powerful
tool of the practitioner to be his unconditional acceptance. With
this primary connection you gain trust and understanding and
then the process of healing can begin at a deeper level. The
release of shame is catalytic – the previous pattern of self-denial
and destruction may be transformed into a higher vibration of
love and courage as the patient no longer becomes a victim of
his past and reclaims his human right to dignity and love. He is
freed to release his pain and move closer to the light.

Practising Creativity

Positive Thought Power

Transform negative thinking into positive power. Begin to praise
and nurture your inner child. Every time you feel a negative
thought rise, cut it short. Imagine you were speaking to a five
year old who had tried his best. Realize you must learn to treat
that child inside you with respect, gentleness and
encouragement.

What you are nurturing is your own self-esteem and courage to try and experience new ways of being and living; you can be, feel and think more creatively.

Worship the God/Goddess Within

Resist the temptation to be negative about your self-image. Remember the inner child! Instead, channel that energy into eating healthily and exercising regularly. Health shines outwards as real beauty. Introduce colour into your life and choose to wear things that make you feel happy when you put them on. Experiment with colour and style, express yourself. Value yourself enough to enjoy the person looking back at you in the mirror.

You are good enough, just the way you are.

Nurture Creativity

Spend one hour a week doing something creative – anything that reintroduces the magic and rhythm into your life. Look back to your youth if you need any tips, or try something new. Choose something that makes you come alive and reawaken the joyful spirit within. Enjoy it – that is the purpose of this exercise, to reconnect with your sense of wonder in creation for creation's sake. Remember, what you are creating is the real you.

Confront Your Addictions

Think about why you may have a self-defeating behaviour or an addiction. Why are you trying to sabotage your future and punish yourself? Are you afraid to confront something deep inside? See if you can meditate on this and let it rise. Sit quietly for ten minutes each morning on waking and see if any answers surface: any wisdom that may guide you to a stronger, better future. Write down any thoughts that may flow from you. Accept what your soul is trying to tell you. Once you have done this you will be one step closer to letting the past go and embracing your destiny. Nothing is more important than your health and self-creation.

Keep a Creativity Journal
~   What would you do with your power if you knew how to handle it?
~   What do you dream of?
~   What would you like to create?
~   What kind of person would you be if you could create yourself from scratch?
~   If you had creative power, what would you create?

Start making plans today and take one step forward every day, even if it's another line in your journal, or another question asked.
Don't fear it, use it!

Remedy Store

Flower essences
~   Billy Goat Plum (Australian Bush Flower) allows sexual pleasure and self acceptance.
~   Turkey Bush (Australian Bush Flower) removes creative blocks.
~   Sexuality is a combination Bush Flower that works well for healing sexual issues.

Crystals
~   Amber warms the sacral chakra, inviting joy and creative energy.
Moonstone balances creativity and divine female energy.

Living a Creative Life
Living with creativity is exhilarating, life-enhancing and life-affirming.
    You are at one with your ability to transform and manifest, like a magician you bring to you what you need. Life is a blast, a pleasure – your senses are alive to music, dance, art and beauty. You see the glory of spirit in every dimension of man's

creative genius. You are completely accepting of yourself as part of life's rich tapestry.

Creativity is separated from the commodity that it becomes in material terms when a critique places financial value on the finished product. True creativity cannot be judged as it has made its own journey. Each piece of work or brainwave has value, be it as a stepping stone to more, or the height of a man's work; they all come from the same origin, they are all born from our spiritual flow and reflected from what we carry within us at that time. Every creative venture tells a story.

We create because we must create and we create without the narrow confines of respectability, validity and value.

We were incarnated to create throughout our journey, to leave behind us mementoes of our life history, the multicolored memoir of our time here on earth. We are proud of who we are and what we are. We play with life, everything is fun and everywhere is laughter.

Creativity elevated with unconditional love fosters self-worth. If you know how precious you are, you will manage to tune out the negative messages bombarding us in our society.

As you find power, flair and balanced sexuality at your core you will not need to be anyone else but you. External limitations of the right clothes, style, figure, weight will appear ridiculous. Health and happiness become paramount. Difference and diversity are good.

You think outside the box and you live with grace and goodness. You were created to create and you will create as long as you live. You cherish every experience handed your way by the universal source and you respect those who are delivered to you to grow with, learn with, share with and play with.

Love is at the heart of all interaction and this Principle guides you in right action in your dealings with others.

You are amazing. You know no shame. You know pride in being you. A quiet inner peace holds you grounded in the blessings you have received. You release old pain with awareness and forgiveness in the knowledge that in that moment you are free to regain your entire power. You are worthy of that power; you are worthy of the dreams that come to you. Watch them daily, water them with praise and encouragement and nurture them with love. One day they may just come true.

The world is your playground.

Creativity

~ Creativity is the Third Principle of Light.

~ Creativity is connected to our sacral chakra, 'The Home of The Self'.

~ Creative power is integral to our human desire to express ourselves and to create.

~ Creativity is linked to our self-esteem and our ability to accept the divine gift of our creative power in all its glory.

~ Creative power is enhanced when we accept ourselves in our current incarnation exactly as we are.

~ Creativity bound with love is beyond judgement; it is a divine energy flow.

~ When creativity is strong we have passion, vibrancy, laughter and a love for life.

~ When creativity is weak we may deny our power with self-destructive behaviour or disconnection from our creative flow.

~ Creativity is a balance of polarities, between the masculine and feminine, hedonism and Puritanism, death and rebirth.

~ Creativity is undermined by shame.

~ Creativity = Pleasure + Personal Power = Procreation.

From a world perspective, we need to remove the taboos and shame that perpetuate the cycles of sexual trauma and addiction, facilitating a universal awakening of self-esteem and dignity.

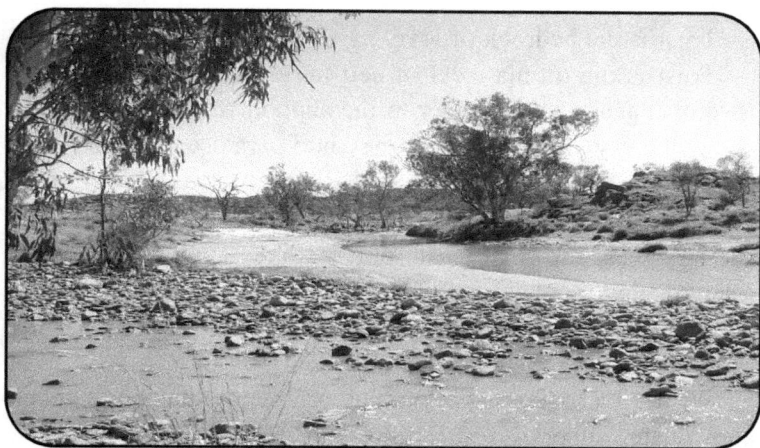

4

Trust

Trust is the fourth Principle of Light. Trust is a choice we all make when we have a faith in the world and what it will bring to us. Trust means knowing what will support you in your growth, what is right for you on your path – trust is what fits you.

Trust is what connects you to the river of Life, a deep knowing that it will be clear to you that what lies ahead is there to teach you what you need to learn.

Trust is an abiding light which moves us from a place of insecurity to one of security, even in hours of darkness when we are blind to see the way, when we doubt ourselves and life's twists and turns.

Trust will carry us with truth to a sanctuary where we ultimately know that the universe wants the best for us; Mother Earth is always there to nurture us if we are willing to accept her guidance.

Trust is the bedrock of love.

Trust is the ultimate act of self-nurturing, when we choose love over fear and surrender to the support of the universe that she will carry you on your journey into paradise.

Why Trust is Important

Trust is at the heart of our choices, intelligence and relationships.

Without trust, we have existence based on fear, which removes us from the ever-flowing energy of love.

We need a basic trust of our environment to interact, connect and relate, otherwise it is difficult for us to open up to opportunities, to mature emotionally or to accept the true beauty that life has to offer.

Trust is like riding the seasons of nature, sensing our own internal rhythms, an emotional wisdom which develops from observing the cycles of life and growing as part of the universal tapestry. It is the common thread that runs in our blood; we are sure we will grow from the seed to the flower to the tree in tune with the passage of time. We rise every morning knowing that this river will see us to the next day and the next and if we allow we will change and blossom and flourish with life as we allow earth energy to impart us with its divine power. Trust is knowing and owning that power, becoming that power and resting in it.

Trust is sureness, completeness and a settled belief that we will be fine.

We trust that we learn what we need to, when we need to and that the experiences that we so deserve will be delivered unto us. Trust is our gut instinct that one path is better for us and we turn towards it: one way will always appear in the light to pull us to it; one way increases our power, all others fade into nothing as they perpetuate fear or limited growth.

~   Trust is self-knowledge.
~   Trust is knowledge.
~   Trust is faith.

~ Trust is belief.
~ Saying I trust you means I believe you.
~ Believing in you means I know you.
~ Knowing you is opening to loving you.
~ Trust must be built in our dealings with one another.

Trust is a pattern of behaviour that revolves around honesty and love. We are not created to give up our complete trust to anyone in an instant, as like animals in the wild we must first and foremost remember the circle of protection that surrounds us. What we trust is that life will guide our way and we continue to have an innate trust in life. True trust comes with knowledge. We are all at different stages in our development; therefore to each other, we may represent a path to be followed, or a path to move past and beyond. What we learn to put our trust in ultimately is the universal source first, and then the choices that support our awareness of what trust means to us. We are not meant to give over our trust without wisdom, as at a certain point in life and learning, we may not be able to act wisely or with compassion to others or ourselves. What should never fail is our internal trust in ourselves to find our path and our trust in the universe to bring relationships to us from which we can learn. If we live with trust we will attract like-minded others into our world to compound and support that Principle; if we still need to learn and develop our instinctual knowledge of trust then we may encounter a few friends on our journey who will teach us a thing or two about the true meaning of trust in a relationship. With trust we are free to be as we are; without it we live in fear and this limits our scope for unconditional love.

The more you vibrate with the Principle of trust the more you will experience the freedom and power of knowledge, support and love.

Authenticity in life demands a truthful expression of who you are – integrity in your dealings marks dignity and great grace. Your path to light becomes paved with gold.

~   I know you tell me the truth.
~   I believe you will not hurt me.
~   I have faith that you want what is best for me.
~   I see you express yourself as you really are.
~   I am certain you will support me in all I do.

How does Trust Develop?

Trust develops from birth.

Our entry into the world as a newborn soul means vulnerability, sensitivity and a complete trust that we will be nurtured, loved and supported. Trust is symbolic of our early relationship with our mother and with Mother Earth. We have no way of caring for ourselves, feeding ourselves or protecting ourselves – we rely solely on the warmth of universal maternal energy to raise us from our infancy. When we cry does someone come to hold us? If we are hungry are we given sustenance? Do we feel safe from harm? Do we feel love, which is the greatest energy of all?

These are vibrations that are laid down in our early matrix, and in later years can still engender a feeling of great fear, insecurity and anxiety when faced with difficulty or challenge. We may not be aware of any kind of surface reason for stress or worry but at the core, if the foundation is not solid, we may still carry a deeply hidden belief that life will fail us in what we need the most. The stress may become such a fixed pattern that it becomes part of our personality so that anything outside logical control returns us to a place of fear – the inner child whose first experience of the world was that it did not give us what we needed when we were scared or vulnerable. A child brought into the world and raised with fear will be sensitized to life's difficulties and will expect the worst until proved wrong. Obviously our thoughts and beliefs colour and attract our experience of reality; as we emit low level vibrations the higher vibrations of love are weakened.

Later in life trauma or setbacks can knock out the Principle of trust and we may never recover the same level of faith in the world if we choose not to heal. Bereavement, fatalities, ill health and relationship breakdowns can all engender a profound sense of loss and an inability to cope with the hand that fate has dealt. With basic developmental trust we may choose to live and breathe again. Without it the path to recovery is harder and steeper, if ever encountered at all. The world remains a frightening and terrifying place, a harsh mother without the warmth of love. The room is dark; no one is there to hear the cries for help.

We all grow and mature and weather the storms of our childhood – the majority of us realize that in time problems solve themselves and for every cloud there is a silver lining. We learn from our mistakes as we grow older and once we have found happiness again our misery becomes illuminated as an education. If we learn to trust ourselves and have confidence in our choices we become attuned to what will make us truly happy and make choices that are for our highest good. We acknowledge that we cannot avoid pain, heartache and difficulty if we are to move onwards and upwards; what does not break us does indeed make us stronger and we become increasingly wise and courageous as we overcome the hurdles and obstacles placed in our way. We discover our true strength in adversity. We know that difficulty only adds contrast to the sweetness of victory at the end of a journey, only makes us appreciate it more. We learn to protect ourselves, trust our intuition and listen in order to guide ourselves with grace and safety – we live without fear – we choose love.

~   It is our choice to choose life.
~   It is our choice to turn away from the darkness and hope to experience the joy of living again.
~   It is our decision to gain control over our mind and emotions and decide to think positively.
~   We feel we are victims of our fate but if we allow our past to dictate our future we are unaware of the choices that lie in

every moment to change the way we think, the way we act, the way we are.

~ We are free to stand above fear and say no.

~ We are strong enough to trust that life will bring us new life.

~ We are always the masters of our destiny.

~ It is a true achievement, once trust is broken, to learn to trust again.

~ Trust in yourself.

~ Trust in your identity.

~ Trust authenticity.

When Trust is Strong

~ We are adventurous, brave, open and powerful. We travel on our path with faith that we will go where we need to go, see what we need to see and learn what we need to learn.

~ We will meet the right people at the right time. We trust ourselves and we trust in our relationships with others. We choose to surround ourselves with others who we can completely depend on as they depend on us to be authentic in expression.

~ We know what we should not trust as our instincts are impeccable. We see clearly that certain avenues are not for us, certain vibrations do not match us and we walk on without attachment or fear that we are making the right or wrong choices.

~ We have no bound duty, we do not act from fear but we act with maturity, wisdom and love that our actions are grounded in integrity and right action. We have trust in our inner wisdom and instincts and let go easily of unsupportive energies.

~ We listen closely to our inner child and heal any experiences that may have weakened trust in our developmental years. We appreciate that to live in fear is not really living and that by working on clearing our souls of pain we give ourselves love and a fresh beginning.

~ We trust our world. We trust that we can take reasoned risks if those risks are right for us, as without pushing ourselves in new directions we will never grow.

~ We have deep and honest relationships with others and also an intrinsic trust in humanity that we are all learning and growing and making mistakes, but ultimately we all need and want the same things: security, acceptance, support and love.

~ We trust in our earth.

~ The vibration of powerful trust is authenticity.

~ The world supports you as you tell the world who you are with pride. There is nothing to hide.

When Trust is Weak

~ We live in fear. Earth energy is blocked, we are immune to the vibrations of trust and love and we cannot believe in the world we live in. We fear one and all; there is no hope, no future, no certainty and no grace.

~ We shield ourselves with our mistrust from ever being hurt again; we shut ourselves away from new and positive experience, new relationships, life and love. We become depressed, lack faith and become angry with ourselves and the world for not finding happiness, but are too scared to venture out and risk losing it all again. Nothing ventured, nothing gained.

~ We may become untrustworthy ourselves, undependable, unreliable, lacking in personal truth and integrity. We don't want people to like us, love us, depend on us, or rely on us. We push love and happiness away because we feel we cannot love, we cannot feel.

~ Our relationships with others are limited and restricted. If you cannot share trust with others you cannot share love as the fear that separates prevents true intimacy and closeness. We may choose people we cannot trust so we never reach a stage of love that opens us up to being hurt.

~ If our trust is broken in a relationship, what was taken for granted is so hard to bring back. Trust is at the heart of intimacy; it gives emotional freedom and is an expression of unconditional love. Saying I trust you means I believe in you, you can be yourself with me, I will not hurt you.

~ When you give someone your trust you are laying a foundation from which to give your love. If you cannot trust you cannot truly love. It is up to you to find that trust in your heart first and then it is easy to open up to love. In the right circumstances trust will be the earth from which flowers of love and happiness will grow until eternity.

~ Once trust is gone, it is hard to believe in the same way. The vibration of weakened trust is betrayal. When your love is betrayed, your love is not trusted. Unconditional love is transmuted to fear and what was solid, honest and true, crumbles into dust.

~ Betrayal is a hard deal to handle; when the one you trust lets you down you are faced with overwhelming emotions ranging from fear, rage, frustration and sadness. When life betrays you how can you begin to find your faith again? If these energies are not released and expressed honestly at the time they can transmute to bitterness, resentment, revenge and hatred. If the party that has been betrayed remains in the same place by concealing or suppressing their true feelings, they will only cause ill health or disharmony at a later stage. It is vital that all issues are dealt with at the correct time and released with love – each individual needs to take responsibility for choosing his own path and remaining true to himself. Sometimes we betray for that very reason, to remain true to a calling or inner voice, and we must accept in each other that we all have our own destiny.

~ Betrayal, if stored within the system or pushed down so that appearances may be maintained, eats away at the vibration of trust, as it will remind you that life has let you down and may well do so again. Betrayal breeds anger and frustration. How can you be free to accept new love and life experience with all the optimism and joyfulness of an open mind if part of you is vibrating with fear and the memory of loss?

~ Release your pain and move on. Let go of what you cannot trust and move on. Trust in life to carry you to a better place if you trust in your essence to be worthy of it. Be trustworthy and attract more trust into your life. Let life trust you to make choices based on love and it will reward you completely.

~ Trust yourself to choose love over loss.

~ Trust in life completely and you will discover that life loves you completely.

Working with Trust

Answer these questions honestly:

~ Do you trust the world?

~ Do you trust yourself?

~ Do you trust your body?

~ Can others trust you?

~ If you answered no to any of these questions why do you think this is?

~ Have you had any traumatic experiences that could have broken your trust in life?

~ Can you think of an exact point in time when you may have lost your faith?

~ Do you worry a lot, or suffer with heightened anxiety, irritable bowel syndrome or obsessive thought patterns?

~ Do you feel you are on the correct path?

~ Are you an authentic person?

Practising Trust

Visualization

~ Lie quietly, light a candle or burn some essential oil. Make sure you feel comfortable, warm and secure.

~ Go back to a time that you can remember made you feel frightened or scared, slowly and gently. If this makes you feel afraid you may want to do this with the help of a friend or a skilled therapist.

~ Can you relive the experience from a place of safety and develop an insight into how this may affected your ability to trust?

~ If you feel a block or numbness you may not be ready to witness the experience so don't force yourself – let it go.

~ If you find it too hard you may choose to write in your journal.

~ If you can understand and see clearly I would like you to clear negative memory in your physical body by sending light and love backwards from the place of safety you sit in now.

~ Imagine a golden light flooding the image and transforming the situation. Try to rewrite your history and complete the story with an ending where all parties understand what has happened, have equal compassion and set each other free to go forwards. Send love back to yourself and promise you will always be there with love and support. See if you can imagine yourself in the present going back to the past and holding the scared and frightened you and transfusing both hearts with love and protection.

~ Maybe you can see fear and pain in the eyes of those that hurt you; by having insight into why they acted the way they did you might be able to forgive and release.

~ Tell your past self that everything is going to be all right.

~ Tell your past self that you trust in the universe to bring you to light. Instruct your higher self and any guides to clear the image of fear and pain and to remove the memory from your karmic record.

~ Release any pain with breath or tears.

~ Sit quietly with your thoughts and trust that life will carry you forwards with love.

This visualization may need to be performed several times to clear the old energy from your psyche and physical body. Using skilled therapists may ease the passage of old fears as well as using specific vibrational remedies.

Don't worry if it does not work for you.

Relax and trust that if you are willing the way will come. If you are ready to let go the doors will open up for you. Be brave, as a life free of fear and distrust is a fuller, brighter life.

Remedy Store

If you are dealing specifically with issues of fear, the following remedies are heaven sent to help release old trauma:

Star of Bethlehem	Releases grief, trauma and pain
Aspen	Anxiety and panic attacks
White Chestnut	For tranquillity when troubled by obsessive thoughts
Mimulus	For known fears

Affirmations

Daily affirmations are essential in teaching your subconscious to reconnect with basic trust. Repeat every morning and evening, seven times. You may want to include some specific statements of your own to clear relevant patterns or anxieties.

~ I trust.

~ I have total trust in the universe.

~ I trust myself.

~ I am willing to release all fear.

~ Everything is going according to plan.

~ Everything I need to know is revealed to me.

~ The world is a safe place.

Confront Your Fears

What is your biggest fear? What would happen if it came true? Would you give up or carry on living?

To be faced with the prospect of this is to have a choice. Imagine how you would feel, what you would do and think.

Visualize yourself being capable of mastering your fear and believing in your innate power and the nurturing love of the universe to carry you through all experience. If this is too hard to do, imagine yourself willing to overcome.

There is nothing to fear but fear itself, and once you have stood up and shot down fear, you are free. We all have the choice to walk down a path to peace, or give in to our fears.

If you have very specific fears or phobias or are dealing with old issues, now is the time to get help and ask for assistance in clearing your pain.

Journal Writing

Write your journal daily and let your thoughts flow freely. It will become much easier to make decisions and choices that support you when you move closer to what you truly want. Writing is a very good way of accessing your subconscious mind and revealing your inner needs.

Authenticity

Present yourself to the world with integrity, honesty, self-expression, clarity and trust in all your dealings. Honour your word and mean what you say. Karma will reward you and the world will soon become an infinitely more supportive and reliable place for you to inhabit.

Living a Trusting Life

To live with trust is to live with the knowledge that we all have the freedom to accept love over fear.

We are all able to look to the light and trust that life will look out for us, no matter what our circumstances or birthright. We can choose to trust life and believe that everything will occur naturally and in order, or we can choose fear. We can choose to seize each day and work on ourselves, to heal old wounds of resentment, bitterness, pain and sadness, and start again.

If we seek we shall find. If we ask for guidance it will be given. If we decide in a moment that we will give up our old ways and search for true meaning, to live with authenticity, the world will support us.

There is infinite power in beholding your rightful place in the world, to stop striving and reaching for that which you are not and accepting the beauty that is you.

If we choose fear we shrink our existence. If we ruminate on our misfortunes, our difficulties, our worries, we forget about all the brightness and wonders our day can bring. We colour our sight with darkness and run from happiness, as we cannot trust that the world has any joy left for us. We will not believe because we dare not believe – we hold the vibration of fear in our hearts and are sure that if we hope for the best our expectations will be cruelly dashed, so it is better to hope for nothing. Our bitterness seeps into everything, turning from the higher vibrations of love and acceptance, miracles and magic.

It is our choice to choose trust over fear every single day. Give trust and you will receive the world's blessings. Become trust and the world will love you.

As you work with this vibration and sense it flourishing in your very being you will experience a broadness and expansion, a sense of rhythm and harmony; everything you need will come to you at the right time, everything you need to know will be revealed and even in times of hardship, difficulty and great challenge you trust that the lessons that you are learning are timely and necessary. You trust that you are one with this flow, you are part of the grand design, that all of us connect and move together on this journey, our karma intertwined. You trust that you will make good decisions based on what is right for you instead of what is good for others. You are clear in your will and path. You stand by your own core beliefs and you become your own beliefs, as you believe in yourself and the world at large.

Trust

~ Trust is the fourth Principle of Light.

~ The foundation of trust is laid in childhood but trauma in later years can easily damage or block the vibration.

~ Trust connects to the solar plexus, which also governs our lower mental energies, gut instinct, health drive and self-identity. This is where we store negative emotional vibrations such as fear, anxiety, anger and resentment.

~ Trust measures our authenticity in this world, our integrity and honesty in self-expression; how much we can trust and be trusted.

~ The opposite of trust is fear.

~ We lose our trust when life betrays us.

~ Fear can be hidden by layers of anger, hatred, bitterness and stress-related patterns.

~ We may perpetuate stressful behaviour and environments as we may hold a deeply seated fear mentality.

~ Without trust we become closed to incoming life energy, the support of Mother Earth and unconditional love.

~ Trust is the bedrock of love and intimacy in all relationships.

~ When we trust ourselves completely we open to greater trust of others in our world.

~ As a universe we have a challenge to push through existing powerful vibrations of fear that threaten to separate us as one brotherhood and fight for greater trust on all levels. When we can open to trust at a higher level we will open to transcendental love.

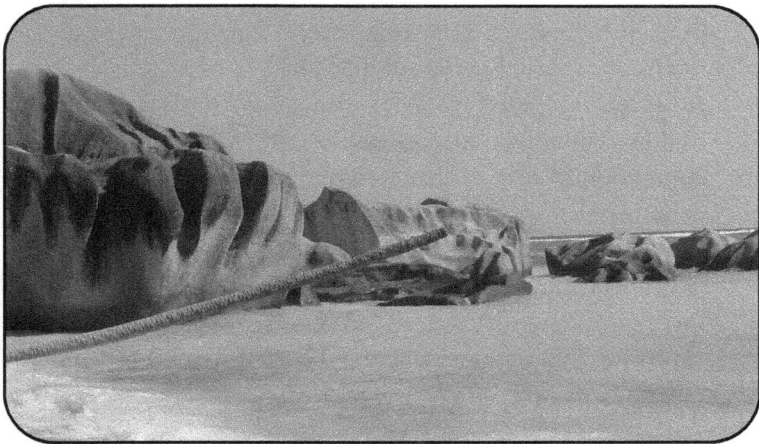

5

Love

~ Love is the fifth Principle of Light, and the greatest Principle of all.

~ Love is an energy that we as humans can all experience and in its highest expression it has the ability to transform, heal, enrich and guide.

~ Love is pure heart energy and has the power to change lives.

~ Love is something we enter this world knowing, it is the very Principle that helps us grow, that enables us to touch each other and connect with each other, and gives us deep meaning in our human existence.

~ Without love we have nothing, without a sense of love in our lives we feel alone. Once we find love within ourselves, we may find love in everything.

~ Love begins with knowing how to love ourselves before we love each other. With the wellspring of love like a fountain in our hearts we can bring forth such tenderness and sweetness that it blesses all that sense it.

~ Love is a blissful state. Love can also be tough, quiet, hidden, understated; it comes in many guises. The expression of love is coloured by the heart through which it is delivered.

~ Love is to give, love is to know, love is to care and love is to grow. We love because we are here to love – to show our love and make our time on earth a happy, wondrous, captivating experience, one that brings joy from sharing this energy with each other.

~ We live and breathe to love.

Why Love is Important

Have you known love? Then you can tell me why it is important.

I believe the soul sings with peace and completeness when we are loved.

If you have not known love yet, then I am sure you know deep longing. Who would choose to live without love? Would their life have meaning if they lived without joy and heart energy? What would we remember from our existence if it was not the rapture of loving a soul mate, an overwhelming, deep, true love between parent and child, the bond that grows over a lifetime between old friends? Love is also a peace that we find in our quietest times, when we feel good about the people we have grown to be and are content in our own company.

But love is more than this. Love as a Principle exalted to its highest expression is known as unconditional love – this love extends beyond our inner circle to a wider, broader feeling that gives to humanity. The love we carry in our hearts, when pure and true, knows only to feel compassion and wisdom. When questioned we will always choose the path of loving kindness, the way of gentleness, complete acceptance of others in our world without hatred or blindness. We accept that to remain true to our Principle we cannot harm or act with malice because our heart will always guide us to act with love.

Choosing to live with love in our lives is a blessing to ourselves, but also a great blessing to the world we live in. Love is like flowers in the heart; when planted they grow into a beautiful garden with the fountain of compassion ever flowing at the centre, the milk of human kindness. We need to keep our garden tended and pull out any seeds of discontent, lest they overrun our garden and make less room for the heart within. We must feel that love in our heart at all times and we must give that love on a daily basis to ourselves; when we have enough love in our lives, when we nurture, protect and give to ourselves accordingly, only then will we have the bounty to spring forth and give to others.

This giving to others, this sharing of the love Principle is what makes our world go round. Random acts of love and kindness daily, synchronicity and synthesis, helping each other on our journey into light carries us all forward on the road to paradise. Together we grow, together we go; onwards and upwards, bathed in the beautiful light of love.

~   Love is an intangible.
~   Love is all knowing.
~   Love is creation.
~   Love is heaven.
~   Love gives life.
~   Love is fearless.
~   Love brings joy, happiness, sweetness and beauty.
~   I love you.

These may be the three most significant words in the world.

How does Love Develop?

I believe that we were all born knowing love.

There is no greater light in life than a newborn baby – I truly believe this power to be the power of untouched heavenly love. A baby smiles and gives the love in its heart. A baby smiles at his mother as she nurtures him and a heart bond is formed eternally. I feel that the heart never loses that capacity to know and share love if it so chooses but over time, if pain is experienced it may become deeply embedded in the heart, preventing easy relations and provoking defensiveness, hostility and mistrust in the nature of love and all it means.

Love is also about the triumph of strength over weakness and remaining true to the calling of your heart. As we mature, if we give up our inner principles to the demands or desires of another we give up our destiny and focus. Do we choose a path of fear over love because it is easier and it fits in with others, or do we stand up for love? If we refuse to align with the voice of our heart we move towards our shadow instead of our light; we move ourselves further from our path. We move from kindness and empathy to disconnection and separation.

Conditioning and cultural beliefs may dictate that we distance ourselves from each other, or that one person is better than another or one way is superior to another, but if we are really honest heart energy transcends all differences between us – we are one world, one love. A child knows no separation and that is his freedom, he gives love freely and openly, is curious and inquisitive – reaps his joy from life from sharing in love energy. We are taught to hate, to fear and blame but if our hearts are taught to remain true and pure our love for humanity spills over as adults and we are able to create lives that are based on an abiding foundation of respect, equality and liberty.

We love and esteem ourselves and we love and esteem those around us.

We let the divine light shine through our hearts to those around us and we experience the karmic return of that heart energy. The more we love the more we know love, the more we experience love in our life the more glorious it is.

If we experience heartache, great loss, disillusionment or mistreatment our heart may close like a flower, too frightened to enter the arena of love again, too tender to allow trust. If our pain deepens or takes hold, this rift can become part of the fabric of our capacity to give and receive love.

We may feel we do not deserve to know love and push it away because we feel worthless. But life will always give love. We may feel bitterness and regret and dwell in our past and what might have been. But love lives in the present.

Our pain may become hatred or fear. We may wreak our revenge on love for the lessons it has taught us. Our heart energy becomes closed or distorted and we have less of a heart when it comes to our dealings with others. We punish the world for what it has done to us. But love comes with gentleness and forgiveness.

We may find it hard to determine who will love us and who will harm us, and find great difficulty in easy expression of love energy in our relationship with others and ourselves. But love will always guide us if we stay open and live with our hearts.

It is our responsibility to discover love and renew our faith in the power of pure heart energy.

Love never gives up on us, even if we give up on it or believe ourselves to be unlovable. Love is endless, and infinite compassion will flow from the universal mother, should we ask for her tenderness. Even in the absence of our blood family or an earthly mother. This energy is timeless, and all around us, should we choose to touch it.

~ Unconditional love is the highest state of love.
~ Unconditional love loves without restriction, without judgement.
~ Unconditional love is a far-reaching love that knows no boundaries.
~ Unconditional love sees the weaknesses and flaws and loves all the more.
~ Unconditional love is forgiving and respectful.
~ Unconditional love accepts wisely and deeply.
~ Unconditional love has faith.
~ Unconditional love is transcendent.
~ Unconditional love is transformational.
~ Unconditional love shows us heaven.

When Love is Strong

You have love in your heart and you brim with joy and splendour. You have goodwill to all men and you love and respect yourself. You smile freely, conveying the blessing of your heart to each and everyone you meet. Good heart energy is warm and cheering, open and true.

You have mercy and compassion for others as they strive to enlightenment and you are gentle with yourself as you journey. In your difficulty and hardship your heart energy will remain strong and offer love at times when your path is uncertain. It will encourage and support without judgement.

Love means loving yourself first and foremost. It means giving yourself your highest good, protecting yourself on your path and providing the right environment for you to feel safe, cherished and blessed. Once you have achieved this you will have plenty of love to give to others. Understanding these principles is vital before we love each other, as how can we know how to treat one another if we do not afford ourselves the same dignity, respect and gentle love we all deserve? We are our own teachers – once we have understood our own needs and boundaries and what makes us feel truly loved it is simple to give that to others: our partners, our children, our friends, in fact anyone we deal with.

How do we like to be loved? We like to be understood, we like affection and honesty, we like reliability and stability, we like enduring deep love that weathers the test of time. In all relationships we like patience, courtesy, respect and kindness – manners may also be an extension of a loving heart. If you expect this from others, first think about whether you are able to give it yourself.

True love is devotional and quiet, very different from the first flush of falling in love or the excitement of a new romance.

True love is solid and dependable, like the warmest, oldest sweater you possess. It may not be glamorous but it will always be there for you, to warm you on a cold night. For you to find this kind of love you need to be ready to give it and find yourself worthy of receiving it. Ask yourself, do you have enough love in your heart to esteem someone highly enough to always care, always listen, and always pay attention to what is really happening? Can you remove any traces of competition, jealousy or comparison to truly want the best for someone you care about?

Can you love with your whole heart?

When you are able to open your heart to this extent, to work on yourself to cleanse the heart of all pain, bitterness and resentment, you will know the true glory of unconditional love and you will reap the rewards of this spiritual power in all its magnificence. You will find love in yourself, love for yourself and love for humanity, for all of eternity. Love will grow and continually spring forth to brighten and comfort you, even in your darkest hours.

When love is strong, you are surrounded by love.

When Love is Weak

When the heart is clouded with past regret, sadness, grief or pain it is difficult to feel the daily joy that love brings. We lose touch with sharing this simple emotion and bringing it out of one another; we forget our own ability to create love in ourselves and to deem ourselves worthy of love from the universe.

We pass our hours in a subdued and lonely state and we feel become shut off from the abundance and harmony in life. We remain in relationships that are based on fear and dependence rather than the free and open vibration of unconditional love; our lives shrinking instead of expanding and blossoming in harmony.

We have little love or respect for ourselves; we cannot look upon ourselves with kindness. We become angry, depressed, bitter and resentful of the freedom that we see others experiencing, but we take no responsibility for bringing love back into our own lives. Instead, we chase it away from us, push good things away as our inner self-esteem deems a certain level of deprivation.

We have already talked of fear as the negative pole of the trust Principle. Most people would name hate as the opposite to love but I would call hate another name for fear and ignorance. It is fear that resides in hearts that cannot love. Hate may develop as a superficial layer above fear, but underneath this strong emotion I still see a lost soul who is frightened of life, who feels life has given up on him and does not love him anymore. This fear transmutes to bitterness and hatred – there is a loss of generosity of spirit and an inability to convey love and compassion to others.

The lost soul may choose to manipulate or play out his inadequacies by causing distress or harm to others. He can only express the isolation and loss he feels within. Hate springs in this state of confusion and suffering – the tortured soul is often the one who tortures others. This is not to excuse the crimes that befall the innocent at the hands of hatred, it is to explain the stem of how an innocent child may have lost the ability to feel and experience love and had to find other ways to survive or gain a semblance of security.

Our world is suffering now – our people are suffering now, too many souls have accepted a life of anger and blame as a way to vindicate the immense internal pain they feel. As a united universal energy, we need to bring forth the power of love in our hearts daily, as love is greater than fear; with love, we may conquer the hatred of man. If we each took responsibility to check our emotional wellbeing, to slow down, to tend to our own needs and treat ourselves with loving kindness, the vast majority of us would be in a better place. From this place, we would be better equipped to send forth pure, loving energy into our world, so we may treat each other with kindness and support. We could give our love to those who do not have the luxury of self-appraisal or self-betterment as they are struggling simply to survive.

As with all actions there is a choice. With all human nature we have a choice. Why bother to free ourselves from old ways, to raise the game, to try and be more loving to others and ourselves? The answer lies in trying it, and feeling so happy with the smallest things that every day becomes sprinkled with magic, laughter and stardust.

~ Loving yourself makes you a worthy and important person.
~ Loving yourself makes you a loveable person worthy of good relationships, experiences, health and protection.
~ Loving yourself means you will take every step to make this happen.
~ Loving yourself means giving yourself life and power.
~ Loving yourself will invite people into your life who will love and support you for who you are.
~ Loving yourself means you can survive alone but choose to share your love with others.
~ Loving yourself means loving the world you live in.

Working with Love

Answer these questions honestly:

~ Do you have love in your life?
~ Do you feel unconditional love for others?
~ Do you love yourself? If the answer is no, why can't you love yourself?
~ Do you feel bitterness, resentment or jealousy towards others?
~ Is there something you are denying yourself that makes you feel envy or hatred towards others?
~ Do you feel angry?
~ Why do you think this is?
~ Has your heart been broken by life or another?
~ Have you healed your heart?
~ What does love mean to you? Where do you source it?

Practising Love

Meditate on Love

Spend ten minutes every day sitting quietly and bringing crown energy to the heart centre. Imagine a golden light glowing from the heart, filling the centre of pure love. If you have a difficult time sensing this emotion, imagine a memory when you felt love or happiness and hold it there. Visualize any dark shadows cleansing and any old hurts healing. Let go of the past and open to unconditional love of the highest order.

Be willing to release all old hurts now, all anger and sadness. Be here in the present and ask your heart to open to love. Grieve for any sadness that is now passing. Ask your heart if there is anything you can to do encourage healing.

Be in the present and try and fully experience the pure emotion of blissful love.

Affirmations

Repeat seven times daily:

~   I open to love.
~   I release all pain and fear from my heart now.
~   I love myself.
~   I am worthy of pure love.
~   I give and receive love easily.
~   I am surrounded by love.
~   Life loves me.

Remedy Store

Flower Essences

Holly	To release hatred and bitterness
Star of Bethlehem	To lift old hurts and trauma
Sturt's Desert Pea	To release deep pain

Crystals

Rose Quartz	Strengthen your heart chakra with this crystal.
Rhodocrosite	Encourages deep healing and cleansing, encourages new growth and fertility.

Cleanse the stone with salt water, charge it with the intent to heal, and place it near you.

Nurture Yourself

Give yourself the love and attention you would give to someone you truly care about. Treat yourself with respect and kindness and listen to your inner needs. Pay heed to the voice of your inner child that may be asking for more of your time and gentleness.

Love yourself every day and keep yourself warm, happy and safe. Spend time with people who make you feel good about yourself and love and support you unconditionally. Once you can do this effectively, choices will become easy. It will become clearer which paths are right for you.

Practice Loving Kindness to Others

This can be anything you choose – just remember to treat others as you would expect to be treated yourself.

Each person is precious, so give them the courtesy and dignity they deserve. Be patient and understanding. Act from the heart. Practise tolerance and acceptance.

If someone does not respond well to your kindness or does not treat you well, learn to voice your feelings with honesty and let them go. Walk away. You need to learn which paths are open to you and which are not; which people match you and which do not. Instead of holding anger and remaining in an unsupportive environment, act with the intent of love and move on. Forgive them if you can and forgive yourself; see the situation as redirection rather than loss. This shows self-respect, self-knowledge and self-love. Move on and keep your heart open. Once you learn to let go of fear and anger life opens up again and delivers to you exactly what you need.

Living a Loving Life

Living a loving life is all about loving life and marvelling in the riches and joy it can bring.

Love is about diving in, taking it all in and experiencing every single minute to its full. Love is about appreciation.

Just as loving someone means you pay attention to them, want to give your time to them, care deeply and try to understand every part of them with a lack of judgement and total acceptance, this is how you should also love life. For what is life but a multifaceted explosion of divine power in all its different colours?

Once your presence is there and your heart is there, life will reward you with blessings and immeasurable reward. It is only when you fear life, turn away from it and refuse to trust it that life caves in, gets smaller.

Open to love every day in every way. Give your love in all you do – if you want to do something, do it passionately, put your heart into it and watch it grow.

Sometimes it is hard to love and you question life and its harder lessons. The pain of existence can threaten to induce such terror and shock that we feel we may never smile, laugh or find peace again. In these moments all we have to rely on is our faith, as otherwise we may doubt that life cares for us at all. If we have patience and courage we will find in time that sweetness can return, and it will be so much stronger, as the appreciation of peace after the humbling experience of loss and difficulty is heightened even more. This is how we grow.

We cannot avoid the cycles of life; we cannot live in fear of our downfall and by doing so prevent life from giving us the wings to fly.

Stay open, stay loving, stay with hope and compassion and belief that life does love you, and will always love you.

Remember to look for the miracles in your life, however small they may be. They will confirm your belief in the constants of life, an understanding that everything does work for the good in the end.

Love those that are dear to you with the whole of your heart – they are the ones that will nurture you in turn and give you an enduring heart centre in your world. Love the things you do and you will reap the reward of witnessing the miracles of your creation.

Be thankful in your high times when you feel you can walk on water – let the memories warm your heart when you push through more demanding passages of renewal.

Be aware that all things have their time and let go with grace and be ready to welcome the new. Feel steady in your heart energy and give your kindness to all.

Most importantly, love yourself. You are a child of this universe and are deserving of the highest, purest, unconditional love.

Love

~ Love is the Fifth Principle of Light.

~ Love is connected to our heart energy and links to our heart chakra.

~ The unconditional love centre opens in a developed heart and conveys an understanding of love as a higher energy extending to humanity and the self. Unconditional love does not judge.

~ The love we give to others is directly connected to the quality of love we give to ourselves.

~ When we have love in our hearts we are able to relate in a compassionate, open and gentle way with others and our world.

~ When love is weak we feel hostility and fear; our hearts close and we become defensive.

~ Deep pain and fear underlie the majority of negative heart energy, including hatred.

~ Our appreciation and love of life correlates with true heart energy.

~ Love is an alchemical power and possibly the greatest of the Principles of light in its ability to connect, heal and change lives.

~ Without love in our lives we become isolated and depressed. We all need love to grow.

~ The amount of love we have in our lives reflects how worthy we feel of that love.

~ Transcendental love energy is a natural spiritual force capable of transforming the way we relate to each other as a universe – if we open to love on a global scale it could shape our future in a positive way for generations to come.

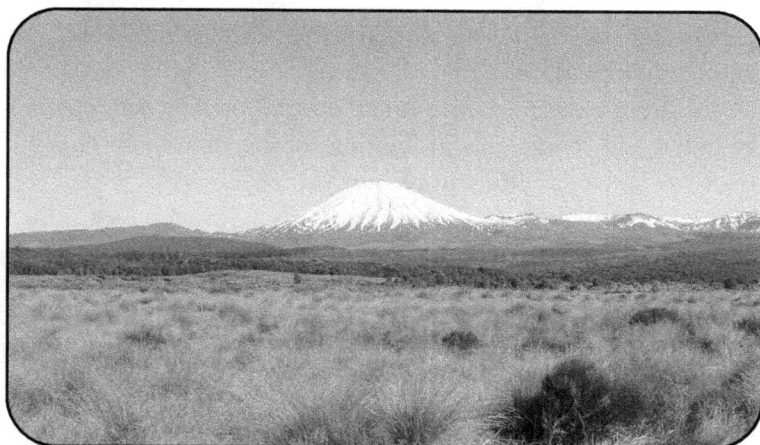

6

Truth

- ~ Truth is the sword.
- ~ Truth is the voice.
- ~ Truth is freedom.
- ~ Truth is the way.

We all seek our own truth as we journey into light for without truth we are lost. We have purpose as we strive for authenticity; we have meaning and self-belief. We want to be open about who we truly are; we want to journey home to our soul essence.

The truth is our story. When we tell the truth others believe in us. When we are honest about how we really feel we believe in ourselves.

Truth is built on honesty, love is built on truth. Truth is integral to how we express ourselves in our essence; if we cannot present the world with ourselves in our entirety we are preventing our light from shining free. Life is the word, our word is our bond.

Confront your inner wishes and desires, dreams and regrets – be brave and courageous in fighting for the right to be yourself without shame and life will reward you.

Be true to yourself.

Why Truth is Important

How do you feel when you tell the truth? Usually it is so easy and natural that it doesn't warrant a second thought.

How do you feel when you lie? Restricted, limited, stifled? One lie often springs from another, and before you know it, you are wrapped in a web of deceit that may have started with a very minor untruth. One path opens up, one path closes down. Or does lying come easily to you, without the twinge of regret or fear of your deception being revealed? Either way, by choosing fallacy over fact we are lying to ourselves – we are choosing a lesser route over a more powerful one, we are choosing darkness over light.

Honesty is part of your journey into light; honesty will help you to be true to yourself and your soul purpose. When you lie to yourself or to another you create a barrier, a wall of defence or mistrust. Your lie falls between both parties, preventing real intimacy or healthy emotional exchange. You may not want to believe the truth will be accepted and so cover up the facts or you may not want to look at reality yourself, too scared to face hard decisions and inevitable actions. You may think lying is being kind – indeed there are situations where you should be sensitive with the truth; but always be honest with yourself about who you are trying to protect.

Lying is a way of shielding yourself from confrontation, loss or change but what really ensues is stagnation, blocking or weakening of the universal force. The powerful beauty of right action is suppressed or redirected and the path that leads closer to freedom and happiness is thwarted.

The truth hurts, but delaying the truth hurts a lot more. Betrayal born of dishonesty is a far greater hardship to suffer than the frank and direct reasoning of a person's heart. To be honest is to be free. To be honest to another is to respect them and give them your full integrity. A man is made by his word and his word will always be remembered. Therein lies courage in honesty and great power in the word.

Trust that time will guide you in revealing truthful information in accordance with the grand design.

How does Truth Develop?

Truth is a medium of self-expression. If a child is raised to express himself freely he will not be afraid to tell the truth. If he is heard he will be used to opening up and relating to those around him in the knowledge that he is unconditionally loved and accepted, whatever he says. If a child finds things tough and knows there is someone who will comfort him compassionately he is not scared to voice his innermost fears and wishes.

Expression is about living in your essence, speaking up but also about being heard and seen. Listening to someone carefully and giving them your full attention is an act of love that nurtures freedom of expression and gives value to what another has to say. Truth will flow naturally and with vibrancy.

If a child is not free to be himself, is asked to remain silent or hide his true self, which is deemed unacceptable, he learns shame and shyness. He feels awkward in company and as he grows older is afraid to reveal too much of himself in case he is ridiculed. He may learn to present a more palatable truth about how he feels, what he is doing and what upsets him as this is easier. Honesty becomes the harder path and lying and acting becomes a way of gaining freedom and acceptance.

This is a pattern that needs to be broken in adulthood as it can hinder intimate relationships and lead to a disjointed feeling of having separate identities or personas. Real emotions and feelings are stifled and it becomes increasingly difficult to own up to what is going on inside. There may be guilt attached to saying what needs to be said; it may be hard to know when to speak out and when to hold back. The heart bears the brunt of unspoken words and grief or anger and burns away at the purity of loving source; an addiction may form, eating, drinking or smoking too much, to distract from the discomfort of holding back or pushing down on the truth.

When the force is scattered the force is not powerful. True power lies in unification. You are what you are and you will do anything you can to be that. When you accept yourself completely others will accept you too.

~ Truth is like a white fire that burns away the dead wood.
~ Truth carves the righteous path on your journey into light.
~ Truth is a power that we wield with mercy and kindness, always aligned with the universal source.
~ We grow in majesty and dignity as we vibrate with honesty.
~ We gain respect as those around us sense an inner greatness, purity and grace.
~ When we are truthful we burn with God's light, for the truth is an act of love that we give to each other every hour.
~ Structures built on false foundations are sure to crumble one day.
~ Those built on love, honesty and spirit will endure into eternity.
~ Truth is the way.

When Truth is Strong

We are direct, honest and judicious with our words. We speak kindly and fairly and harmonize our voice with our heart and wisdom energy.

We find it easy to modulate our emotions and rarely use our words to hurt or find fault. We listen equally well; with karmic return this means you will be heard. We use our voice to express our truth – we give of ourselves freely and we sing and laugh with the joy of living. We communicate easily with others and pass on information, as we obtain learning from others.

We are guided easily on our path as we share with others. We believe in ourselves and are comfortable being ourselves at all times. We feel free to speak up or be quiet when necessary and feel no restriction.

We choose people that mirror our confidence in self-expression so we may be truthful and open in our dealings. We know ourselves well and take full responsibility in our life to take care with our actions, knowing that self-discipline gives us ultimate freedom.

We are empowered so we have little need to blame others, as in our power we are able to change the course of our path instead of relying on others to do this for us. We know that by telling the truth we are giving ourselves the greatest gift: the courage to be seen exactly as we are. We understand that truth is like a sword: cold and hard, but effective and clearing.

We know that truth is timely and we choose to share our truth with others when the time is right. We use it wisely and understand that truth is subjective. Your truth may not be my truth and your truth in ten years may be very different from your truth now.

We spare the truth when our heart asks us to be gentle, or when we see that the truth would further no-one. Truth is the warrior's way.

When Truth is Weak

The voice is expressed from the vocal area and remains disconnected from the higher faculties and the heart. Thoughts and emotions may be felt deeply and strongly but without the voice to express them they become bottled up and stifled. The heart carries emotional pain and loss but the mind may also become frustrated and anxious as the truth of the matter becomes confused and blocked.

The soul is desperate to be heard and released but the words are stuck. It is vital to speak up, to put that energy across, otherwise how can anyone else react to you. They may sense emotional change subconsciously but we all need to hear each other to truly understand. The voice may sound overly quiet, fast and furious or hold bitterness or anger – the truth is being distorted as the throat chakra is not able to let go, to spring forth to harmonize in melodious speech or laughter.

When a person hides his truth he is hiding from life, he is pretending to the world to be someone different. There may be several payoffs for lying: to remain in the same relationship, job or position of 'safety' a person will lie to himself that everything is okay. If there are difficult memories or traumatic incidents in the past that have never been revealed or worked through, these too are pushed away and the throat is sealed over. If we don't want to tell others the truth to protect ourselves from confrontation we lie. In fact we lie whenever the need takes us.

Why shouldn't we lie? Because it takes from life, it limits our freedom and movement through life, it holds our power back. Lying to others is thoughtless and shows a lack of respect for others in our dealings. We become less authentic people.

Who wants to rely on a liar? Who will believe in someone who cannot tell the truth? You may say you get along just fine telling the odd white lie and indeed there are times where we are forced to tell a 'version of the truth' to make a social situation easier, but on the whole pretending forces you into an emotional plane where you become increasingly restricted and are less likely to attract honour and grace.

Some people lie about themselves because they find themselves unworthy; a lack of self-esteem creates a real sense of inadequacy and they feel that elaboration makes them more acceptable to others. Or they may lie for the sole reason of pushing others away. Dishonesty stems from a lack of self-love and integrity; if you don't feel you deserve love exactly as you are, you may attract situations where you cannot be faithful, loyal or true to those you love. You let people down first, lie to them and make them see how unreliable you are so they cannot love you.

You need to feel you deserve love before you claim it as your own.

Don't be a pretender; be honest about who you are, where you came from and what happened to you – however difficult this may be, the people who love you when they know everything about you will always love you.

When you find a person who really loves you, treat them with respect and give them all the love in your heart.

Working with Truth

Answer these questions honestly:
~ How honest are you?
~ If you lie, why do you do it?
~ Is there anything you are lying to yourself about?
~ Do you have any secrets that you are scared to confront?
~ Do you take responsibility for your life?
~ Do you feel free to do as you choose in life?
~ Are you shy; do you find it hard to express yourself?
~ Were you heard as a child?
~ Do you listen to others?
~ Do you communicate with respect and kindness? How could you improve this?

Practising Truth

Dealing with your Truth
If you have been hiding something from yourself or others it is now time to confront your secrets and take responsibility for bringing them to the light. Take power over them instead of allowing the opposite to continue.

Seek therapeutic help and access the hidden memories, bring them out and set them free. They do not belong in your heart or your mind any longer. If they remain there they will continue to cause anguish and disharmony and a whole host of behaviours that serve to distract you from the inevitable reality of what is done. Look them in the eye and say goodbye. Make the changes that will make you happier and set you free.

Acknowledge the wonderful things in your life right now and accept your current truth.

Look forward and plan what kind of truths you would like to see flower in your future; see your essence running free.

Learning to Listen

Pay attention closely when someone speaks to you, when they tell you their truth. Watch yourself and see if you are truly hearing them or if you are thinking about all sorts of other things. You are giving that person your love and respect when you listen closely. You are allowing them to express freely and move along their path.

If you can really honour those you meet as you journey they will honour you. There may be a time when you truly need a friend and the universe will deliver as you give a little of your patience and compassion. To be heard can be truly cathartic; just the act of sharing a problem or secret that has weighed heavy for too long is enough to make things a whole lot easier. A child may be frightened or worried and may need the reassuring voice of a trusted adult to make him feel safe again. Lend your ears with love.

Use your Voice Wisely

Try to be responsible with your words. Speak kindly of others and try not to gossip or backstab. This energy will come back to haunt you. Don't take out your anger or frustration on innocent bystanders. This is your stuff; take responsibility and deal with it. Use your words to laugh, sing, relate, entertain, caress, educate, communicate, heal and embrace. Use your words positively and truthfully. Be compassionate when you slip but keep up your own standards. Check yourself for dishonesty and bring yourself back to an authentic level.

The more your words harmonize with spirit, the smoother your journey will be. Do as you would be done by. Words can harm, punish, hurt and wound. The memory of cruel words can live a lifetime and damage irreparably. Be free with your expression, but speak from the heart. We can all be more gentle and sensitive with each other.

Remedy Store

Crystals

~ I highly recommend working with crystals to unblock a sealed throat. A mixture of energy techniques may be used: either lie with the stone on your throat and visualize it clearing the blocked field, or wear it on a necklace or ring or put it near your bed as you sleep. Make sure you soak the crystal in salt water overnight and charge it with the intent to heal. Try a turquoise, lapis lazuli or any of the beautiful blue gemstones; they are all brilliant at clearing the throat and improving expression and assertiveness.

Flower Essences

~ Bush Fuschia (Australian Bush Flower) enhances expression on all planes.
~ Southern Cross (Australian Bush Flower) taking responsibility.
~ Larch (Bach) will improve self esteem and self expression.

World Truth

Who can you trust?

No-one, it seems, in this day and age. Our politicians, our media, our businesses – it appears just about everyone is lying. It is a wonder we have faith in anything or anyone anymore – do we even expect ourselves to tell the truth when the perceived standards in society appear to fall so low.

We have little control over the paths of others. What we can master is our own behaviour and actions. We have the choice to stop lying, start telling the truth and speaking up; we can lead our lives wisely and compassionately. Dishonesty is rife and embedded in many industries as a way to amass money and power; this mentality may exist in many planes of life but not in the higher realms and vibrations where true magic takes place. You can take a stand by doing a daily meditation on honesty and truthfulness and giving full appreciation to the gift of freedom that is our birthright. We are free to express ourselves as we are born to be. We can choose to forgive others who are still learning the rightful way and still create an authentic life.

In many countries children are not raised with freedom and honesty, women and men do not have liberty or freedom of speech. They are not heard, their wishes not respected, their personal responsibility is taken from them. To live without freedom is one of the greatest crimes against humanity, and one that diminishes and weakens. Let us use the freedom that we take for granted to empower humanity and to shift the axis of free will and liberty from dishonesty and oppression.

Choose now to act with honesty and responsibility, align yourself with the light.

Living a Truthful Life

There is no greater freedom than truth. The truth will free you.

Sometimes it is hard to accept the truth about people in your life, or a situation you are in; you may be afraid to confront the truth because of the consequences it brings, and the changes you will have to make to your life. But if you don't do it, you are living a shadow of a life; you are building the four walls of your prison.

One path leads to unparalleled beauty and joy as the new life you build is set on secure and firm foundations; the other path leads to a life of 'safety', and involves fitting in to others' expectations and needs and squashing your soul into a role that is to be expected, that in reality makes no-one happy.

If you are brave enough to take the leap from pretence to authenticity, the world will reward you, but you have to take the first step. Once you step out of your box you will be greeted by a world where it is safe to be exactly who you are. You will meet like minds who do not hide or suppress their individuality but who are attracted to the mighty of spirit and pure of thought. By taking this first step you are saying to the world that you are ready to take responsibility for your life, you are ready to own it, cherish it and love it. Your rewards will fit the magnitude of your bravery as you can only move closer to your path of right action as you refuse to act with dishonesty any longer.

When you lie to yourself you are lying to those around you. Your soul is restless and cannot settle or commit easily because it is in the wrong place.

Once you are free to move towards your truth and you accept it as your rightful due, it will be easy to love, to build and trust in others. Making decisions will come easily.

When we tell the truth we vibrate with spirit – it feels wrong for dishonesty to come from our lips – it tastes wrong, it feels wrong, we cannot digest it.

There is always a path of truth if you go with the way.

When things are frightening or confusing, remember to remain as honest as possible and ask to be shown a way. When truth is in your bones you become a trusted power. You raise the universal vibration and you lift away from fear. Fear makes us lie, fear makes us pretend, fear makes us mistreat others. Fear takes away from love. We feel the need to protect ourselves, think only of ourselves because we cannot trust.

Give yourself truth and you will find yourself resting within a safe haven, an oasis of calm.

~   You have nothing to hide.
~   You are what you are.
~   Your truth is enough.

Truth

~ Truth is the sixth Principle of Light.

~ Truth vibrates from the throat chakra.

~ Truth is intrinsic to the expression of our essence.

~ Truth is powerful when we are completely honest with others and ourselves.

~ Truth is diminished when we lie, or pretend with our words or actions.

~ Truth is a gift of love that we share by honest and respectful dealings in our world.

~ Dishonesty is the opposite pole to truth and moves us further from our path.

~ Truthful action leads to great freedom.

~ Our words are powerful and we should use them with wisdom and compassion; they have the ability to harm as well as heal.

~ Telling the truth aligns us with spirit and keeps us close to our path.

~ Listening is a mark of respect and by karmic return allows us to express ourselves openly with others.

~ We must continue to strive to raise the world vibration to one of truth and honesty by refusing to live our own lives in darkness.

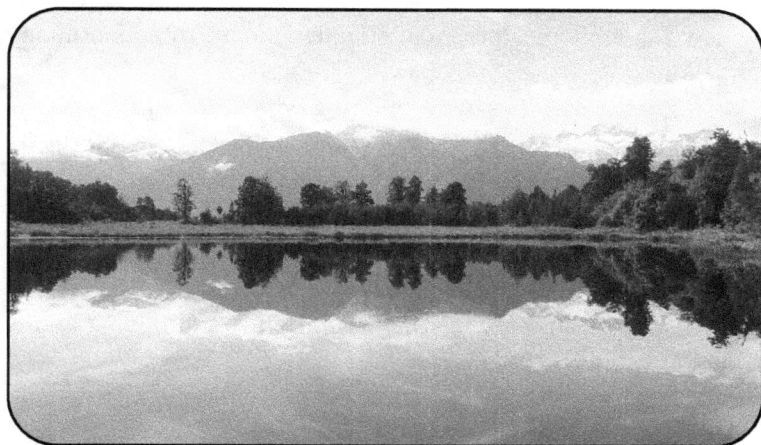

7

Wisdom

Wisdom is the seventh Principle of Light. It opens the doors to perception. Wisdom is knowledge deepened with the compassion of the heart. Wisdom is not afraid to see the total truth and accept it for what it is. Wisdom makes decisions and choices in alignment with The Way and universal law.

Wisdom is the sage we have in all of us, a sense of knowing without knowing why, a sense of seeing without our eyes, a sense of guidance on our chosen path by using the gifts we are given to bring us closer to our divine mission.

The sage sits quietly, observing all and saying little. He notices much of what goes on around him because he keeps his own counsel and develops his own strength of judgement and intuition instead of relying on others to lead him. He knows that in his quiet meditation, he has at his disposal the insight of the heavens, which will always give the best advice; the way of right action that embodies the most effective course of action in any situation.

This is the Master's Way, of doing without doing.

Wisdom comes to all of us if we stop to listen or call for help. A message will come in some shape or form, an answer or a sign, if we stand still amidst the confusion of daily living and have patience; if we have the courage to accept the truth of any problem and make things happen for ourselves.

Wisdom means carving your own destiny and relying on the inner voice that we all carry to sail us to safe harbour.

Wisdom leads us away from danger like an all-seeing parent, taking us from difficulty into the haven of light.

Why Wisdom is Important

Wisdom is necessary in life to help us realize our destiny. On a daily basis we need to make intelligent choices about all manner of things – the outcome of these choices will determine how the picture of our lives ultimately looks. What do we want? Can we think carefully about how we may achieve this? Can we make clever decisions, take all the right actions, pray for guidance and follow the signs to help us manifest our heart's desire? Are we wise enough to know what is right for us and what is wrong for us? Are we thinking logically or intuitively? True wisdom is a mixture of both.

Wisdom in action often means being brutally honest with ourselves, and not being afraid to see the harsh reality of our past, present and future. If we hide from what is really happening in a job, relationship or family dynamic, we are hiding from taking positive steps towards our own happiness. If we do not want to see the difficulties we will never face up to them. It may be easier to brush them under the carpet for the time being but sure enough, the tricky bits of life will come back to bite you. Turning a blind eye to negative situations merely delays the inevitable and holds you back on your path.

Wisdom is seeing everything and then taking practical action. Wisdom is about taking a path that is right for you, but this may involve letting go, creating a new life or starting again. Wisdom also helps others in their distress, never taking the lead or forcing a plan but gently showing a light at the end of the tunnel, options, solutions and reassurance in times of need.

Wisdom is gentle and noble, clear-sighted and honest. Wisdom is willing to learn. Wisdom is prepared to make decisions, take chances and understand, as it is divinely insightful. Wisdom leads the path to inner peace.

Are you ready to be truly wise?

How does Wisdom Develop?

Wisdom is learnt at the school of hard knocks. Wisdom may be carried through from our previous lifetimes. Wisdom is also learnt by experience, growth through pain and love, and by our chosen life teachers as they enter the schoolroom of our current incarnation. Wisdom is learnt by making mistakes and discovering that one way works better than another. Wisdom develops by picking ourselves up and starting again, knowing that this time we will take better care of ourselves.

As children, we become wise as we absorb hundreds of different concepts daily, eager to learn and progress. We are encouraged by our earthly parents to keep trying and keep going, and praised with each small step we take. When we remember the positive process of learning we are keen for more. If we are scolded for making mistakes or not being good enough or quick enough as we learn we may cease to try, believing we are not worthy of true success as we will never be good enough. We put undue pressure on ourselves that anything less than 'perfection' is useless. Aiming for 100 per cent in every test is a sure-fire way of creating performance anxiety in even the youngest minds – no-one can be perfect and we should not expect ourselves to be. Nature is not designed to be perfect, we are beautiful in our triumphs as well as our losses – it does not make us a failure if we lose, we are winners for trying. In fact it is the very process of trying that engages us with growth and maturity, over the end result of winning. It is the trying that hones us, the grace in difficulty, the process of reaching up and becoming more. If a child is accustomed to thinking he is stupid, useless, lazy or any of the other negative putdowns that poor teaching or parenting conveys, that child will grow into an under-confident adult with a perception that he is unable to make the right decisions in his life. He will doubt his own wisdom. This inability to think clearly for himself often leads to dependency on other people's advice or will; he will be crippled by a sense of poor judgement and connection with his own intuition and logic. Destructive criticism is cruel and heartless; it saps energy and drains self-esteem – a young plant finds it hard to grow without nourishment.

However academically smart we are we all have the ability to know ourselves.

We do not need a degree to learn quickly and become skilled once we are on the right path. It is all about finding that path and everything just falling into place. We all can be good at something if we want to be. Every child has a talent and something that makes him unique.

We are all quite able to think for ourselves and to guide ourselves with our wisdom throughout life's ups and downs. We are all able to learn from the past and perceive clearly what appears before us if we want to. We may choose to give up our wisdom and allow others to make those choices for us, as it is easier than believing in ourselves or taking responsibility for the actions that transpire from our insight.

We are all wise in God's eyes; we all have access to divine knowing and guidance, should we choose to open our eyes.

Wisdom and the Energy Field

Wisdom corresponds to two of the upper chakras, the forehead and the ajna chakra. The ajna sits in between the brows and is the seat of intuitive wisdom, knowing and the collective subconscious. We sense and perceive our surroundings and have access to a vast amount of information through this chakra: our past, present and future lives, our memories, dreams, hopes and fears and patterns and data that match the signals and information we are receiving every minute. We use our eyes to pick up visual stimuli but it is with our ajna chakra that we really see. When the ajna becomes highly developed the third eye, which hovers just above, may open, which increases our psychic and subtle faculties and may accelerate the inflow of additional information.

Students of the higher realms may work hard to see with the third eye, but I would say we are all quite capable of seeing with our deeper senses if we begin to trust our intuition more, and rely on our instincts about people, places, symbols and synchronicity. Once we believe we have these powers, our insights will broaden and deepen as we awaken a part of our brain that we have culturally forgotten. We see and perceive so much by just being around another's field – the words that come out of that person's mouth are just part of the equation – how did you truly feel during the interaction and what did you come away 'knowing?' This knowing faculty is underused but you can sense when your instincts are triggering your thoughts and, depending on how comfortable you are with the message you are receiving, you may act on it, ignore it, shut it away for later, observe it or block it.

Our forehead chakra sits above this and processes our logical, practical and rational thought, common sense and dissociated clear thinking when faced with a problem. It formulates plans, solutions and actions and when functioning well it keeps our minds clear and sharp, with the ability to rapidly take decisive action when necessary without confusion or hesitation. For true wisdom we need both of these energy points to be working together like a team, balanced and interconnected, each one of equal importance.

In our current society, I often see an imbalance in favour of the forehead, as in our modern world we become distanced from our intuition and do not know how to trust our instincts and knowing. The forehead becomes enlarged, arrogant in its dominance, science overruling faith, the paternalistic preference of logic and rational calculation overriding the feminine sense of deep wisdom, symbolism and subconscious messages. The ajna becomes squashed and eventually defunct and the patient loses the ability to sense subtle guidance and signals regarding his own destiny. He will in time feel lost and disconnected from his soul wisdom, his perception becoming flattened into a single plane of black and white with little contour or contrast. The opposite occurs very occasionally, with a tendency to rely heavily on emotions and feelings without the common sense to ground the information into logical action or sensible and relevant steps. As human beings we need both sets of skills to be wise. We need to use all the available information at our disposal and then act on it in a clear and precise manner that works in our favour. If we choose not to see clearly or to block our deeper wisdom we are often making choices without the full facts and may find it slower and harder to walk our rightful paths.

~   See clearly.
~   Think peacefully.
~   Act kindly.
~   Live wisely.

When Wisdom is Strong

We see clearly, we see deeply and we act wisely. We want to see the truth and we are not afraid to handle the information we receive with respect.

We have compassion in our perception of others and are slow to judge as we realize we are all learning in our current incarnation.

If we accept the truth about others it frees us to decide whether we want a connection with this person or if it may be wiser to walk away and give them the space to work it out. In this action we give others the permission to do the same and there is no need to be caught up in relationships where we blame and criticize each other's faults. If we choose to stay then we must search for unconditional love within our hearts and accept as we find. We do as we would be done by.

Judgement is corrosive and limiting – how can we know what is really going on in another person's heart and soul and believe we may treat them as we see fit if what we perceive does not please us? If we feel strongly, it is our responsibility to act in a manner that benefits others and ourselves; we do not use judgement to cause harm, meddle or hold hatred against others. We see and we act with right action at all times. When we choose wisdom we colour our judgements of others with love – we realize for every mistake there is a lost soul who has lost his path in some way. If we make snap judgements over another person we are choosing only to see the negative, and by karmic return we are inviting judgement upon ourselves. So goes the saying, 'Never judge a man until you have walked a mile in his shoes.'

We seek the truth at all times and we look for love in all situations. We treat ourselves lovingly and make decisions based on what would bring joy and nourishment to our inner child.

Wisdom asks for self-discipline; we often need to let go of what no longer serves us and the forehead chakra will give us the basic and honest facts of a situation if we are willing to see them. If we can honour the calling of our internal wisdom we will walk a path of peace, self-knowledge and strength of character as we stand by any decision that is seated in love and integrity, even if it means standing alone. Our wisdom cannot accept falsehood and if we try to fight against it we will become ill, our soul will sicken and we will develop a host of symptoms and signs that originate from imposing false control and suppression of our true nature and beliefs. The truth will always out and our wisdom must be respected.

We know what we know and we generally know deep down what we need and what we must do.

When wisdom is strong we are secure and calm. We are flexible, quick and supple in our thought processes, and we keep an open mind to all possibilities. We trust our own judgement and do not rely on others too much for advice, but also know when we need help and support and are not afraid to ask for it. We are fair-minded and compassionate in our logic, and are willing to educate and inform ourselves for the benefit of others and ourselves.

We guide as we are guided.

We have willpower and strength of character and have as firm a hand over our thoughts as we do over our actions, as it is our thoughts that breed our actions.

A healthy mind means a healthy body and soul and we feed ourselves daily with positive encouragement, love and good faith.

When Wisdom is Weak

We are confused and scattered, doubtful, cynical and scared. We worry incessantly and doubt our own ability to find the light.

We feel the world has failed us so we put little credence in the earth's ability to support and guide us. We find it hard to think clearly, make decisions or accept the truth.

We do not want to see the truth of others and we would rather shut our eyes to what our own wisdom is telling us. We may quite literally develop short- or long-sightedness as we struggle to equate our worldview with our soul wisdom.

We feel negative and think negative thoughts; we may be self-destructive and critical, passing unfair judgement on others and ourselves.

We may be rigid in our mentality, unable to open and soften to different concepts. We may find it very hard to accept another's point of view and remain dogmatic and arrogant in our logic. This occurs when we feel threatened – if it is not our way, and our way only, how can we validate ourselves as worthy? These souls may have been told as children that if they did not get things 100 per cent right, they were stupid and therefore unlovable; so they have to be right. There is a lack of security in self-worth, an inability to admit, 'I don't know', 'I could be wrong', 'there is so much I can still learn'. There is fear that by making a mistake, forgiveness will not be granted.

Naturally we are all entitled to our own point of view because that is exactly what it is. We all see a situation from a different location and look down on the same point from a very different standing; in each case, we are all bound to see the world differently even if we are all looking at the same thing. This diversity in perception is a beautiful thing and should not be forced into conformity – instead it brings richness and colour and magic to our world. If we were each given the task of making a short film of our world experience they would all be different but each one equally valid.

If we give credence and permission to democracy of thought, in turn we give ourselves the freedom of unilateral self-expression and uniqueness. As we journey on our path and gain experience our world view changes and we must permit these changes to occur as we develop as humans – as we are flexible and gentle with our own process of deepening wisdom and maturity so we must be sensitive to others on their path. We all need to learn and make our own mistakes in our own way. If we enforce a way of thinking or value system on another, this splitting of the mental faculties between the soul reasoning and the projected system may create grounds for mental illness.

Stress occurs when we overload our systems, take on too much or push ourselves too hard in the wrong direction without the nurturing guide of compassion for the self. Depression occurs when anger is internalized and turned inwards and the ensuing negative patterns of blame, guilt and self-negation take hold; the patient would rather hold his emotions within than express his anger healthily because he cannot or will not take responsibility for his feelings of resentment, frustration and betrayal. OCD (obsessive compulsive disorder) occurs if a superficial system of control is imposed when the internal mental/emotional world is in chaos. Panic attacks and anxiety take hold when trauma or sadness are internalised instead of being expressed. If a lid is put on anything, the system will

eventually blow – if a psychological rationale is imposed on the
soul by the person or by another's will this discrepancy between
the soul truth and the altered state will cause dysfunction of the
mental faculties and disorder of logical thought and reasoning
and intuitive wisdom. Madness is the soul's cry for help. I
believe psychotic disorders may occur when the soul is so
shocked it chooses to live in an alternate reality and abnegate
responsibility in this life. Living in this world may be too painful
and choosing to hallucinate or experience a delusional reality is
preferable to facing the starkness of a loveless and frightening
world. The protective shields around the upper chakras, ears and
eyes may be ripped apart and the patient experiencing altered
consciousness may be truly experiencing lower astral energies
and life forms.

Using excessive drugs or alcohol may temporarily or
permanently open the doors of perception for good or for bad. If
we are lucky we may perceive the upper realms, and the visions
we receive may enlighten us on our path – unfortunately if we
are not careful we may fall prey to negative energies which are
around us all the time but we just don't see because of our
protective shields. Tearing the protective layers of our auric field
can lead to a loss of grounding, security and sensibility as we
become exposed to additional and unnecessary influences.
Alcoholism and drug addiction can lead to a path of mental
unrest and persecution if the habit is not released and the energy
boundaries are not restored to full health. It is our responsibility
to check our health and to keep our minds clear, pure and strong,
as when we vibrate with clarity we are able to access the greatest
energy of all – spiritual bliss.

When wisdom is weak our spirit is scattered. We move
slowly through life and find it hard to harness the energy to
make our plans become actions. We procrastinate because we
doubt ourselves and we are fearful and hesitant.

Fear clouds our vision and judgement; we are negative about
others and ourselves. Fear buried in our psyche colours our
future actions, limits our choices and makes us wary of life.

Prejudice originates in fear and ignorance; misunderstanding breeds hatred. It is so important that we perceive each other clearly and with love, and that we accept each other with complete tolerance. If we do not understand something we should never be too humble to ask and to learn. If we do not understand somebody, we should try and think why their behaviour is as it is. A lost and lonely child is usually at the heart of most bad behaviour. What we hate in others we often hate in ourselves and we project our shadow outwards instead of taking the time to learn a little more about ourselves and sending love to the parts of ourselves we deem unlovable.

Once we can accept ourselves we can accept others; once we love ourselves we can love others. We are all the same at heart; we all need to be looked upon with gentleness and compassion. Put your wisdom to good use by getting to know yourself better; the key to true wisdom lies within.

Working with Wisdom

Answer these questions honestly:

~ Do you trust your own judgement?

~ Do you trust your intuition?

~ Are you quick to criticise or pass judgement?

~ Why do you think this is?

~ Do you make decisions easily or do you rely on others excessively?

~ What do you dislike about others?

~ What do you admire in others?

~ Can you relate your projections to the inner workings of your own psychology?

~ Is there anything you are afraid to accept or see in life?

~ How would your life change if you perceived the truth in every situation – what actions would you need to take?

~ Is your soul truth aligned with your world view?

~ Do you find it easy to realize your goals and dreams?

Practising Wisdom

Check your Thoughts on a Daily Basis

Purity of thought leads to stillness of the mind and happiness –
we are all able to master our thoughts instead of being a slave to
them. We forget that our daily reality is defined by our world
view, and we can choose to be positive or negative. With
positive and loving thought we experience a broadening and
sweetening of our life experience and this rebounds to us a
hundred fold as we send that positive energy out to others. We
are protected karmically in this way, as if we refuse to judge
others, we become more universally accepted and respected.
Choose to be broadminded when seeing others in your world
and you will find it easier to be more forgiving of your own
weaknesses. Cut the blame, criticism and self-doubt and reach
for compassion, understanding and tolerance.

Be Willing to Accept the Truth

Open your eyes to the true story that lies in every situation and
make your decisions based on clarity over confusion or lies.
Your life will become easier as you choose to confront your
demons. Try and understand more about yourself and others and
bring to the light everything previously hidden. It is time to let
go of outdated perceptions and base your choices on your
newfound wisdom. If you are scared of the inevitable truth you
are blocking your path ahead: you will experience anxiety and
unease as you are grounded in fallacy rather than reality. The
truth will lead you to your destination.

Remedy Store

Bach's Flower Essences

Scleranthus	For indecision
Wild Oat	To see your path clearly

Crystal Therapy

Amethyst	To aid spiritual awakening
Celestite	To align with heavenly wisdom
Fluorite	To clear and harmonize the mental faculties
Clear Quartz	To stabilise and balance the upper chakras

Essential Oils

Geranium	To calm and balance the thoughts
Rosemary	To aid concentration
Clary Sage	For euphoric wellbeing
Orange	For joy and positivity

Meditation

This is a powerful practice that draws in spiritual light energy to cleanse the mind, body and soul, and connect with spiritual wisdom. It helps to heal any existing imbalances, reduces worry and gives peace of mind. It is best practised by sitting cross-legged with a straight back on a rug on the floor, or sitting upright in a chair. The mind is stilled and focuses either on a single image, a mantra or a counting rhythm related to a slow, regular breathing cycle. You can imagine and feel the energy running up through the spine to the crown; from earth to heaven and back again, as the mind is steadied by the breath. After a few minutes' meditation, your thoughts should become clearer, and tension and stress should dissipate as you increase your connection to source.

When practised regularly, this connection with the divine eventually supercedes earthly anxieties as the higher vibrations raise the power of the mind. With time, you should find greater energy and poise and find it easier to make decisions as you flow with universal wisdom.

Affirmations

Every negative thought can potentially be changed to a positive one. Write your recurring negative patterns down and begin the process of changing your mental plane to a nourishing peaceful and loving environment by eradicating damaging and destructive thought forms. Eventually your conscious mind will accept the change after your subconscious mind has processed and put in place the new positive message.

Keep a Straight Head

Caffeine, alcohol and drugs can provoke depression, anxiety and fear in the withdrawal stage. You may be using these substances to deal with your worries through escapism but be aware that the clarity and precision of your mental faculties may be overlaid with the energetic force and nature of these substances.

Clean up your lifestyle and find peace and stability in your daily patterns. Cutting addictions may be a challenge at first but as time passes you will appreciate the value of seeing and thinking clearly.

Psychotherapy

Examination of your patterns with an experienced therapist can open doors to your soul that you never knew existed. We can all journey inwards and aim to heal the wounds or learned behaviours that form our shadow. Once we have accepted ourselves with love we may accept others and we will find our path blessed with love. Insight is the key to healing and by perceiving our blocks we may surpass them as we see them for what they truly are – a mere thought form.

We all strive for inner peace and by working with ourselves to make our inner landscape a welcoming and loving space we have a strength we can return to time after time on our journey. If you do not want to or cannot talk to another person now, try journal writing every morning and look for self-therapy books which will unlock these doors and provide valuable insights into why you do the things you do, and how fear or the past may be holding you back from your true potential and divine mission.

Living a Wise Life

Wisdom grants you special powers: the power to see within, the power to decide clearly on the right course of action, the ability to predict potential pitfalls or trouble on your path and the eyes to watch for signs and symbols that will guide you safely on your journey.

With true wisdom, we are perfectly aligned with divine wisdom and our knowing is charged with spiritual light. Our choices are heavenly choices, we act with others and ourselves at heart, and we can only move in the flow of the right way.

When we cannot see we ask for help, when our road is blocked we trust the universe is blocking us for a reason.

We are wise with the experience of living and breathing the universal design and our intelligence is boundless as we capture the collective consciousness channelled through our own energy field and prehistoric neural networks. We sense through a million channels rapidly and multi-dimensionally – we may trace a person's expression and know in an instant what he really means. Whether we want to accept this truth is another matter – what we choose to do with this information is another choice again. When we are truly wise we never block this information – we become infinitely wise the more we allow ourselves to learn. With our heart and mind we then decide on the right course of action and constantly ask for guidance to protect and lead us down the path of right action, every day becoming stronger, wiser, calmer and braver.

A man will not become wise by hiding from the truth, nor will he become wise by using any information he receives to deleterious effect. He becomes wise by respecting and trusting his wisdom and maintaining a compassionate and fair mind at all times. He remains wise by remaining humble, as even in his wisdom he can never know everything; otherwise what would there be to learn? Learning is pure joy in itself. Learning symbolizes growth. We remain wise by remaining students of life and humanity and by being ever interested and fascinated in what the world has to offer and the stories that people have to tell. I am constantly amazed, touched, saddened, uplifted and educated by the tales I am told by my patients – we all have a past and we can all teach each other from the tableaux of our existence on this earth.

We are here to learn and unite and we are here to teach each other. We invite each other in to bring us challenges so we may grow and shift and change and overcome. Those who you conflict with are trying to teach you more about yourself. Instead of blaming or judging, think carefully about what they might be showing you about yourself. What could you improve to deal with this, what could you change in yourself for the better? Once you blame you hand over your power – we cannot change another but we can always change ourselves. Once we have reached the wisdom of our challenge this person will cease to be an issue and a teacher – you may give your thanks in peace and forgiveness and move on. You have grown.

Choose wisdom, choose life. Open your eyes and see the true glory of our world. Go out there and take it all in; learn, see, do, think, act, communicate, believe. As your wisdom rises, so your vibration increases in frequency and the doors will begin to open, not only to our earthly realms but also to the heavenly ones. Protect your fields from the lower astral planes and reach for the upper dimensions and prepare yourself to be profoundly and infinitely amazed. The world will never look the same again and your world view will not only encompass our world but our universe, galaxy and beyond. Be brave and be wise and your courage will be rewarded. For what greater reward is there for true wisdom than the company of angels who were always with you but you were too blind to see?

Wisdom

~ Wisdom is the seventh Principle of Light.

~ Wisdom relates to the forehead and ajna chakras and true wisdom involves a harmonious and balanced functioning of the two.

~ Wisdom is accrued through the lessons learnt through life experience.

~ Wisdom is knowledge tempered with the compassion of the heart.

~ Wisdom guides and leads us forward with right action.

~ Wisdom helps us to make decisions easily, plan effectively and gives us the gift of foresight as we learn from past experience.

~ Wisdom is weakened when our mental energies are blocked, scattered, imbalanced or confused.

~ Our doors to perception are opened and we are increasingly willing to see the truth of the world around us.

~ Wisdom foregoes judgement as we try to understand each other with tolerance and respect.

~ Wisdom is aligned with divine wisdom and guidance is readily available should we seek answers to our problems.

When our soul wisdom is suppressed by projections from others or an enforced self-imposed belief system we become mentally ill.

We have the power to master our thoughts and send out positive, loving vibrations over destructive, negative patterns.

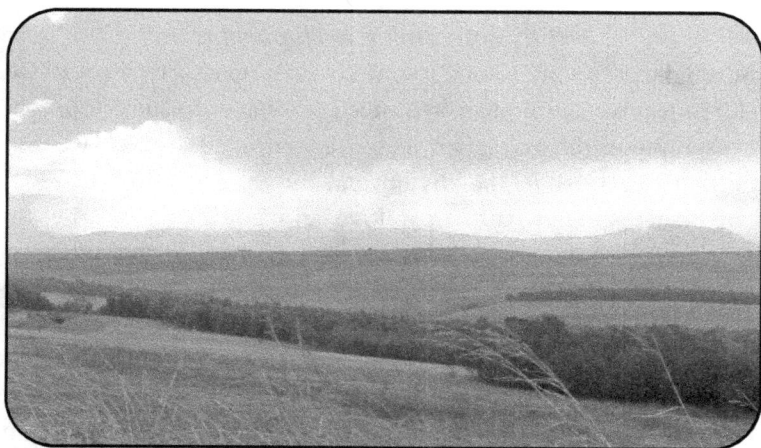

8

Surrender

Surrender is the eighth Principle of Light. Surrender is the golden crown we wear when we reach our utmost potential and rise to the glory of incoming spiritual light.

We surrender to the great and mighty, we put our absolute faith in the heavens and we align ourselves as part of the grand universal energy. We rise to the godliness we all carry within us.

We give up our egos and submit to something greater, we stop pushing and struggling and settle into the flow of life. We take time to appreciate the little things, the beautiful things, at each step and walk hand in hand with our destiny as divined by our answered prayers.

Surrender releases us from the eternal struggle. Surrender acknowledges complete acceptance. Surrender shows ultimate trust in ourselves and the earth that we will be guided onwards to our rightful place.

Why Surrender is Important

Surrendering to life is an act of faith but a necessary one. As we surrender we relinquish the need to have to perform, get everything right and effectively see into the future. We are putting our trust in the divine and as we give that trust the universe responds with great love and guides us effortlessly where we need to go, creating the exact situations that we need to learn from in this life.

When we seek to impose too much control over our environment, lives and the people in it we are saying that we do not trust that our needs will be met. By letting go and believing that what we need will come to us at exactly the right time in the best possible way we are stating that we trust the world to love us and support us. We relinquish our fears in this moment and empower ourselves to release anxiety and worry. The energy released by setting aside fear is then best spent to further manifest our dreams. There is alchemy in absolute surrender; our fear is transmuted to love.

Fear is the barrier that pushes away our goals; it breeds stress and disease and encourages expenditure of an awful lot of power that could be best spent productively. Fear may in fact manifest our worst nightmares as the sentient consciousness is diverted from hope to what we most dread. Fear overshadows attainment of our goal; the soul sees the opportunity to overcome fear by learning and our goal is pushed further into the future. This is why we must remain detached from the outcome. We forget the immense power we harness in our minds to create our reality and instead of expecting the best for ourselves we expect the worst. We could use that energy to grow, to experience more of life, to laugh and have fun, instead of worrying and fighting against life spiralling into a cycle of draining negativity. When you choose to surrender control over events you are taking a positive step towards happiness. When you give up, life often picks up and shows you the way when you could not see. With objective distance from a situation, possibilities appear clearer. Often when we want something so much, it is because we internally fear that we shall not be given it. Taking a step back and losing attachment to the outcome allows the energy to flow freely once more and allows you to deal with why you felt so afraid in the first place. Something may not be working for you right now, something may be blocked; accept this, take sensible steps to seek support and find a new way, then release your wish.

Surrender is the final admission. Surrender declares that we must find the light to guide us through difficulty. Surrender states we are eternally and divinely linked to our path.

How does Surrender Develop?

Children are especially good at surrendering. They are entirely dependent on the universe to support them and if nurtured correctly will continue with an innate belief that they will always be cared for. They are brought up to expect that they will be sheltered, fed and loved and as they grow older the quality of their early environment will dictate how secure they are with the fundamental belief that the universe will provide abundantly.

If childhood is tough for physical or emotional reasons, such faith in life may be scarce and a normally placid child may remain hyper-sensitized to loss, danger or failure. If something occurs that destroys the sanctity of the early environment, the child may grow into an adult who has a deep suspicion of what life will bring. This may be quite evident in behaviour patterns, ability to commit to things or relationship dynamics. It may be experienced, however, on quite a subconscious level – if life doesn't turn out as expected a disproportionate anxiety reaction may occur, associated with depression and fear for the future. It is then hard to believe that things will turn out okay, even though this may just be a rerouting or redirection by the universe. Because of previous events, this experience becomes a mirror of early loss and a reminder that life is not to be trusted – just when things were levelling out life may come along to trip you up. This cynicism needs to be weeded out, as it serves no-one and creates a gloomy landscape in the mental/emotional body. Anxiety levels may lie dormant but as soon as a challenge appears the old fear rears its head and creates ripples of stress and worry throughout the energy field. The connection to the divine may be open but the negativity detracts from pure faith and provokes a feeling of continuing vulnerability and insecurity.

We all experience loss and pain and, at times, feel grief and sadness; this is life's story. Pervading fear and anxiety, however, prevent us from enjoying and appreciating the wonderful things we are given every day. We fail to see the beauty in our lives or stop to smell the flowers. We remain on tenterhooks, awaiting the next disaster to befall us instead of making the most of the time we have. Surrendering to crown energy means accepting the twists and turns of our life in their separateness and being prepared to move on and love again with spirit. Surrendering to the journey means we open up to the highs and lows and accept them for what they are, but we never stop having faith that life will continue and we will experience joy again.

Surrender.

~   We are all part of a bigger picture.
~   We all flow together.
~   We are all connected.
~   Everything happens for a reason.
~   There is timing in everything.
~   Everything you need to know will be revealed to you.
~   Pray to the divine.
~   Open your crown to the white-gold light.
~   May spiritual bliss guide you.
~   May you commune with your guides and angelic helpers.
~   Their words will comfort you with gentle encouragement, forgiveness and complete acceptance.
~   Find faith and your faith will carry you.
~   Find faith and your faith will restore you.
~   Find faith, and may you find enlightenment.

When Surrender is Strong

We feel connected, guided and protected. We feel integral to the universal energy and rarely feel isolation or loneliness, even in our quiet times. We are sensitive to the signs in our lives and pay heed to the messages we receive all around us, and every day. We trust ourselves to make the right choices as we feel we are constantly guided by right action. Right action brings us closer to our path, makes us calmer, happier and stronger and promotes positive growth in our lives.

We know that everything must happen in accordance with the flow of life, as a river runs, as growth must occur in order to allow us to flourish in the best possible way. We sense that the universe does indeed want the best for us even when we are blind to see it.

We send our wishes and desires out into the universe and then let go of them, knowing our prayers will be answered at the right time.

We have faith, especially in difficult and troubled times, as it is then that we are carried by our sense of a greater power.

Letting go means letting go of grief, letting go of old ways, letting go of everything that seeks to hold us in one place, because ultimately we must move on and continue to live and breathe again no matter what happens.

Our faith strengthens us from within, it is our torch in the darkness, heaven beneath our feet, love in all we do and appreciation for every good thing that we experience. The more we meditate, the greater our connection to our spiritual source, the more we will know complete power and knowledge of the way and our path. The more we let go the freer we are to let go of our ego and the confinement it imposes on us by its expectations and limitations.

When we surrender our ego will to divine will, it is far easier to achieve soul happiness and harmony.

When Surrender is Weak

Our nature is controlling and limited. The crown is shut down and little divine energy enters. Existence becomes limited to what the ego demands and needs, and energy is expended on answering those demands, whether or not they are healthy or efficient.

Without source energy entering there is little sense of a bigger picture or a feeling of harmony with spirit or the universe. As there is no trust in the divine flow there is a sense of isolation and an increased need to regiment life and impose strict rules and discipline to ensure plans go ahead. We may appear outwardly successful, but our internal emotional life may be strained and pressured, as there is little incoming support or guidance from the crown. Alternately, we may be incredibly chaotic emotionally whilst our external personality is obsessive to a fault, trying to exact some semblance of order in a disorganized world. In both cases, we could do with the energy of the crown to enable us to let go and let ourselves be guided and nurtured by our access to spiritual power and love.

Letting go is a hard thing to do – letting go and relinquishing control over your environment; but without the presence of this faith, the resulting stress can jeopardize any sense of inner peace and contentment.

When surrender is weak, we are always fighting the world, always expecting it to fail us, completely separate from the knowledge that it is there to connect with us and guide us.

We procrastinate because we fear we do not have enough within ourselves to make things happen instead of realizing that by working with the divine we will be shown our path.

We all have divinity within us; by exploring this part of us we open a door to a greater level of understanding, communion and freedom. Even if we have no faith in God or spirit it is useful for us to realize there is some higher energy that connects and flows between us all, that is responsible for a sense of synchronicity in all our lives. If you cannot find spirituality, be willing to acknowledge that the world is on your side.

Working with Surrender

Answer these questions honestly:
~ Do you worry a lot or suffer from anxiety?
~ Are you controlling by nature? Do you deal with change or the unknown easily?
~ Do you feel isolated or alone?
~ Do you believe that the future will bring you the things you need?
~ Do you have a sense of your own spirituality?
~ Do you feel connected to the rest of the universe?
~ Do you feel guided?
~ Are you in touch with your own spiritual helpers?
~ Are you good at letting go of the old and welcoming the new?
~ Does your ego drive you or do you flow with divine will?

Practising Surrender

Meditation
Meditate daily to increase your spiritual power and purify your crown energy. Sit in silence and focus on a white-gold light at the crown. This light connects you to source energy and enhances your personal power by realizing the energy of the higher realms.

Over time, this practice will improve your sense of peace and wellbeing and if done every morning will stay with you for the rest of the day, putting the general trials of daily living into perspective. You will soon begin to realize you have the ability to rise above your daily troubles and start believing that a greater force will come to your aid and guide you to good.

There are many ways to meditate - you may repeat a mantra, visualize a single object such as a flame, or just be in stillness as you raise the energy from the base of your spine to your crown.

Remedy Store

Crystals

~ Amethyst
~ Celestite
~ Snowy Quartz

All these crystals will improve your spiritual connection and development if used for meditation or healing.

Homeopathy

Potencies of amethyst and celestite are available from good homeopathic companies. These remedies clear lower energies from our crown chakra, promote calm and peace, and increase our connection to heavenly light.

Letting Go

Make a note of the things you try to control – people, situations, appearance, the future.

Instead, think about what would make you happy, what would be your ideal outcome. Your current level of thinking may not find a path to your goals but with universal energy on your side you may be shown the way. Make practical notes based on a loving heart and see if you can start to implement some positive changes. Then let your wishes for a predetermined outcome go; let it go.

You cannot control another person's destiny, you cannot change the way they are, so let go of any hold you may have over them now. Retrieve your spirit. Let go of outworn patterns and dynamics, anything that is not working. Let divine energy heal you and move you forward. Let it help you access the truth and take you further down your path.

Control originates in fear – we may not want to face the chaos, so we control. We may be frightened of the truth, so we impose order. Take a deep breath, acknowledge your pain and work through it – accept divine wisdom and let go.

The Grand Design

Start trusting in the bigger picture. Watch for coincidence and look for deeper meaning in what you might be learning. Watch for timing – do you think the universe may be helping you by arranging things in a certain way? Look for blocks – did this mean you had to take a different direction that worked out better in the end? Ask daily to be shown the most effective way to create or do something and ask yourself honestly if you are finding daily life easier, smoother. Let the universe help you with your dilemmas.

Try not to blame yourself when things don't work out – there may well be a reason that we cannot account for until some time has passed. If something difficult happens which is saddening or unexplainable, remember your faith and realize this is also part of the grand design. With light comes darkness, with joy there is sadness – this is the duality of life and nature and we will all at some time in our life experience great gain and great loss. This is what makes us who we are and this is what carves our soul. Our faith and our spiritual connection will always lend us succour in these times and help us to remain close to our path on our journey into light.

~ If life is especially hard, ask the universe to carry you.
~ Sense synchronicity.
~ Believe in serendipity.
~ Reach up and touch the cloth of heaven.
~ Wing your dreams down to earth.
~ Live in enchantment.
~ Glory in the powers that be.

Surrendering to Life

Release and relax. Let go. Once you achieve complete surrender and flow with your environment instead of controlling it you begin to live a life of faith over fear.

Faith wins and you start to believe in the masterpiece that is humanity, feel a part of the universe, become one with the great energy that is our cosmos.

Letting go of your ego energy and choosing to move past this brings you closer to the soul, deeper and nearer to the wishes of your inner child – in alignment with what would make you truly happy.

Look within instead of outside of yourself. Bring your focus to your own happiness instead of the lifestyles of those around you. The ego loves to compare and find itself wanting.

Dream your dreams and set them free – watch them come back to you as they fit perfectly into the overall plan with harmony and grace. Your guides and angels will sing for you with beauty and love and ensure great tidings will dawn on you as they see fit, in time and in order.

Everything must happen in a certain way for it to be built on firm foundations. The truth is strong and indeed timeless and will not bend and break in an instant, but for this to be borne out it must be grown in harmony with nature's way; first things first.

Deadlines are desires imposed by the ego – they stem from 'I want'. Deadlines set the soul up to fail, leading to despair and a confirmation that things don't always work out the way you want. Instead, let go of those pressures and believe that the universe will deliver to you at the right time, in the right way for you to be loved in the best possible way.

The universe needs you to deal with certain things first for truth to bloom and blossom in your garden of love. The universe would like you to remove the blocks you carry with you internally, the fears that prevent you from fully partaking in and enjoying life.

The universe needs you to know that as long as you care for and love yourself first it will support you and nurture you endlessly and undoubtedly. This is the meaning of faith.

If you have faith you have life. If you choose to look at life in this way you will soon understand that the complexities and intricacies of your life all fit as perfectly as pieces in a jigsaw puzzle. The blocks you see preventing you from taking a certain path will point to a new direction. The significant events in your life came about with a resonance in your soul as if they were destined. If you reach out, what is right for you will come to you. If you trust your intuition and the messages you receive you will be eternally guided. If you take heed of warnings and move gracefully and gently through life you will be protected. If you value yourself and love yourself truly you will accept greatness into your life and let the universe love you.

Surrender now to love and happiness, surrender to the will of the universe, which sings with the sweetness of your divine soul; open up to the heavens and let their light shine down on you. Believe in the grandeur and glory of the powers above – you may dwell in this perfect bliss every day of your life if you acknowledge its wisdom.

We are more than members of the human race, we are deeply spiritual beings, and in this exaltation so we may find our righteous path.

Surrender

~   Surrender is the eighth Principle of Light.

~   Surrender is connected to the crown chakra.

~   We receive divine spiritual energy through the crown and are connected to source through this point.

~   Surrender aligns us with our soul wisdom and removes our ego consciousness.

~   Surrender asks us to remove control from our lives, and to find faith in divine guidance.

~   Controlling our external environment originates from a deep fear of life and an intrinsic belief that it will let us down.

~   Forced control and an inability to accept the truth about our environment or relationships can result in anxiety and mental illness.

~   Imposing deadlines and restrictions on our lives sets us up for failure so we may relive a pattern of a disbelief in faith.

~   Surrender is the greater Principle, as above fear, we find faith and are able to see the bigger picture.

~   When we surrender, we flow through life.

~   When we truly surrender, we are able to accept guidance from our intuition, spirit guides and angels, and divine wisdom.

~   Letting go of fear and finding faith in ourselves, each other and our universe is the biggest task we will ever need to achieve.

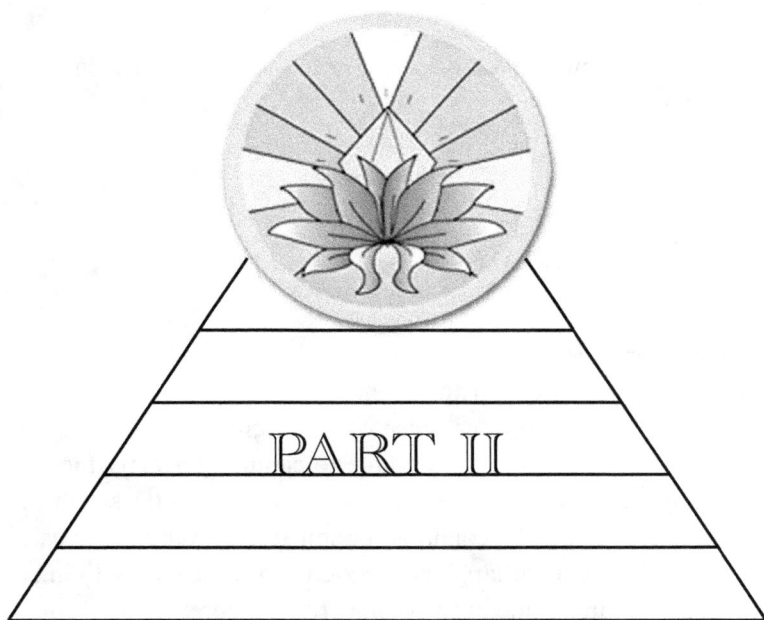

PART II

The Higher Soul Collective

The Higher Soul Collective comprises the final four Principles of Light.

~ Peace
~ Karma
~ Forgiveness
~ Unity

These Principles are intuited as high frequency vibrations, attuned to incoming spiritual light.

When we develop our sense of conscience to align with the universal light source, we are able to capture perfectly the true meaning of these Principles, elevating them effortlessly in our existence. We become conduits for spiritual power and we carry this into the world at large as an extension of heavenly living.

Their nature is fine, refined, unearthly, ethereal and infinitely beautiful. They intimate how mankind can learn to live as one in harmony, overcoming the heavy earthly vibrations of pain and fear.

We are able in our current incarnations to bring divinity to our world, and peace and happiness to our souls, by opening up to increasing amounts of spiritual love, and surrendering to the divine wisdom guiding us along our path.

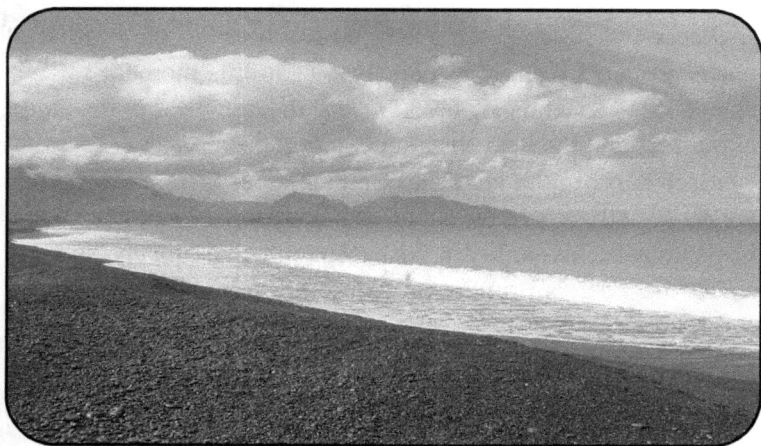

9

Peace

Peace is the ninth Principle of Light, and welcomes in the final quartet of higher vibrations.

Peace marks the entry of spirit to soul, where consciousness meets the crown. This is an indefinable point where God energy transmutes with material energy and connects us to heaven.

With peace, we are in complete harmony, we move and rest in equal measures, we feel no resistance as we grow closer to cosmic universality. We are still in chaos and powerful in the knowledge that we are always at one with God.

We feel no fear; we release all expectation, and indeed we have no ambition but to move closer to our soul purpose, for therein we find truth. The hardship stops, the regret and sadness fade away, as does the eternal search for even higher highs with the inevitable lows.

Peace has no contrast, peace just is.

Peace is where we are quiet and can listen to the beating of our heart and we smile to ourselves as in this moment we feel splendour and rightness, and we sense the greatness of the world at our feet and the heavens at our fingertips.

Each part of us is alive and happiness becomes knowing that we are exactly where we should be, and exactly who we should be. With peace in our hearts we accept ourselves deeply, and find solace in receiving guidance and comfort from divine source. We put one foot in front of the other, moving surely and with certainty, ever closer to the light.

Why Peace is Important

Peace represents true happiness. Happiness is peace of mind. Peace of mind is feeling and knowing that everything is as it should be. Peace is the gateway to heaven on earth.

Knowing that everything is just right means we can live without fear and live in our power. We are supported in our endeavours and guided in our daily actions.

Without fear in our souls we open completely to love and trust, and receive more from our universe than we could ever imagine. We are rewarded with the light of God as we step forwards into his cosmos. When we reach upwards into the higher realms, climb our mountains and realize this is where we always belonged we are enlightened, protected and held. We are safe. We can stop pushing, striving, comparing and grasping, and be still in our acceptance.

Happiness is releasing to love and opening to peace. Great happiness can really be appreciated as peace after a time of great turmoil.

A life half lived is a life half won; to feel joy we must have known sorrow. To truly appreciate happiness as a neutral vibration rather than a peak is to have struggled with difficulty.

We will not find happiness in a shop window; we find happiness by living a daily life of harmony, our thoughts and emotions blissfully serene.

As we listen to our lower vibrations we are filled with comparison, negativity, inadequacy and emptiness; we counteract these messages by wanting more and more, appeasing our ego demands and searching for goal fulfilment that stretches our sights above what we are and also above the other mortals we share our world with. We need to have more, be more and be seen to be more. We lose connection and synthesis and become stranded as we separate. Life is not a race or a competition.

The ego demands that we are greater and better, that we must be more than ourselves to love ourselves. We lose the peace of gentle compassion in our search for outward success.

All journeys lead to greatness if they are borne from truth. If we are guided by love we will eventually become what we are destined to be and we will find great happiness in accepting that for ourselves as there is immense power in acknowledging that we are enough.

To purify a heart and soul and offer love to all we meet is a grand achievement; to lift our spirits to the sky and pray for the good of our fellow man is a miracle.

Working with Peace

Answer these questions honestly:

~   Do you have peace in your life?
~   Is your mind free and untroubled or do you worry a lot?
~   Do you place undue pressure on yourself or feel that a lot is expected of you?
~   Do you feel you are enough exactly the way you are?
~   Do you feel you need to be a success to be worth something?
~   Do you feel aligned to you soul purpose?
~   Are you happy?
~   If not, why not?
~   What is your idea of true happiness and peace?
~   Does this mirror your life as it is now?

Practising Peace

Write a Life Plan

~ With a pen and paper at the ready, sit in meditation for ten minutes and connect with source. Ask for guidance with this task.

~ When ready, write as quickly as you can, what would bring you true happiness in your life.

~ What does happiness mean to you? Be honest. This is about your soul and not your ego – this is about peace instead of status.

~ What would help you to experience true bliss and bring your day-to-day life closer to heavenly living?

~ Write freely and when you have finished look closely over what you have written.

~ Are you able to make some of these dreams into reality? Take your first step today and remain with source.

~ Remember, happiness is always balance and happiness is where light and dark meet in harmony. Happiness is not to be found at the extremes of life but as a daily blessing. Happiness is a constant where everything is as it should be.

~ Seek to remove the obstacles in your life that are preventing you from achieving true peace of mind, either by physically changing some aspect of your life or by emotional acceptance and inner growth. Introduce more of what makes you happy and see the balance shift.

Find Peace

Try and experience peace and stillness of mind every day, in your own way. Find your sanctuary and let it still your mind so you may receive divine guidance easily and clearly.

Find a sacred space where you can clear your mind of the daily grind and reconnect with who you are on the inside.

Silence is golden.

Manifestation

Visualize or draw your deepest desires and send them to the heavens.

Write a wish list to the universal source and sign it and date it, then put it away. Ask for help in moving closer to your wishes. Release all fear and flow with the timing of the grand design. Put your trust in the universe that it will deliver the right things to you at the right time.

You may wish to make an image board with drawings or cuttings depicting your dreams; ensure that you can look at it daily. This will impact on your subconscious and help guide you on your path, reminding you of what is important to you.

Health

Your body, mind and soul need to remain in good working order to retain balance and flow. When the energy body is functioning harmoniously, divine energy will flow inwards easily. Pay attention and correct any minor problems quickly. Respect your needs. Minimize your intake of substances that unbalance the natural energy flow, those that induce an immediate high, usually followed by a low. Sugar, alcohol, caffeine and drugs may give you the kick you crave, but if overused, will impede your mental and emotional stability.

If you are using them to cover up a problem, try and find a solution, or someone to help you through this.

Ultimate happiness comes from peace of mind.

Meditation

Use your sacred space to connect to the incoming source. Cleanse your mind with the source light, contact your guardians for guidance and call your spirit back to the present.

As you wish for safety and blessings send your divine blessings outward so others may benefit.

World Peace

Can we attain world peace? Do we want to attain world peace? Does man actually enjoy suffering and fighting? Can we ever imagine that man will release his ego and open to love for the good of the universe?

Some of us truly want this for our future generations. Some may not believe it will ever be possible. We can but hope and dream and strive together, for herein lie our salvation.

Pray for peace, do your bit, send love to those that need it and be slow to judge those who are slow to learn. We are all at different stages on our journey into light. We must accept the weaknesses of others as we accept ourselves but always have faith in the goodness of man.

Dare to keep believing that one day, we can all change, we can all be better, and that one day, we may all live as one family.

Remedy Store

Crystals
~ Celestite (gemstone) channels heavenly energies.
~ Black eyed Susan (Australian Bush Flower) reduces anxiety and striving.
~ Serpentine (gemstone) enhances calm and connection.

Living a Peaceful Life

Everyone searches for happiness. In our current times it has become the 'holy grail' in our existence. In our 24-hour culture we can have everything material we want right now, but true happiness may elude us. We may be looking in the wrong places.

Our media portrays happiness as an aspirational state defined as having all the necessary symbols in our perfect lives so we may be perceived as 'successful' people. The world of advertising purports that to be seen as a success by having all the relevant attributes equates to a blissful existence. This drip-effect of imagery is pervasive and insidious, so that over time we may fail to see how we can achieve happiness without the perfect home, car, clothes, figure, family, number of children, job, friendships and generally fabulous lifestyle.

Happiness is not a measure of achieving these external material markers, but a sense of self-knowledge and love for yourself, the individual you are as you stand alone, naked of any attachment or possession. Happiness is a skill. Happiness is replete in a life that is closely aligned to the needs and wishes of each individual soul and inner child and a willingness to put those needs first bar any outward pressure or expectation. Happiness can be learnt. What this comprises is different for everyone – we each have our own paths. To nurture ourselves to an oasis of protection and acceptance is to achieve inner peace. Happiness is a stillness of the mind, an awareness of love in our lives and an excitement and joy in continuing our journey in accordance with our own personal truth and freedom. Happiness is contentedness; happiness sources energy from fulfilling self-actualization and earthly work.

Peace is the pleasure derived from rising above the restrictions of expectation and comparison and finding solace in your own singular life and a connection with the divine that allows us to relate to people in our world with compassion and humanity.

Man's will becomes merged with divine will. Divine will wants only what is best for the inner child that resides within. Divine will wants us all to live with truth, harmony and sweetness. Divine will create lessons for us all so we may learn to love each other better and make our world a better place. Divine will sends us countless blessings as we fulfil our soul mission here on earth.

In peace we are able to notice the small treasures that life brings us every day. We are eternally sustained by the wonder and beauty around us.

With a turbulent mind, we are distracted by our worries; our fears draw us inwards, we become increasingly preoccupied and blinded to life around us. We fail to see what is really going on.

We have chosen to shut out the light and to sit in a darkened room alone.

It is time let go and open to peace. It is time to be still.

The questions are: do people actually want to live without pain and fear? Do we actually really want happiness? Once we let go of our pain who are we? Where do we go when we have no-one left to blame? What is on the other side of darkness?

Happiness and true peace can be even more frightening than fear. We are empty and we are one with divinity. We are free and released from duty and regret. We can do anything we want to. Can we then accept that we need to do nothing? Can we relinquish control and begin to flow? Can we accept that in our peace and stillness we are enough? Can we simply choose to be? Can we love ourselves in our communion? Can we love ourselves when we feel nothing more than quiet acceptance, humility and grace? It's a brand new experience, untried and untested.

To release all the negativity and find enduring happiness you may be surprised by the lack of fanfare, the absence of intensity, the wide open spaces of heaven on earth.

This is love. Love accepts you exactly as you are – you can stop trying now and start living. Peace is found when we are happy to be with ourselves. There are no secrets any longer. We have stopped running from the things that trouble us and have released then into the ether. We have stopped trying to be other than what we are. We are great but we are humble. We are equal. We deserve complete peace and happiness and we give ourselves up to this.

~   Peace is silence.
~   Peace is stillness.
~   Peace is acceptance.
~   Peace is light.
~   Peace is beauty.

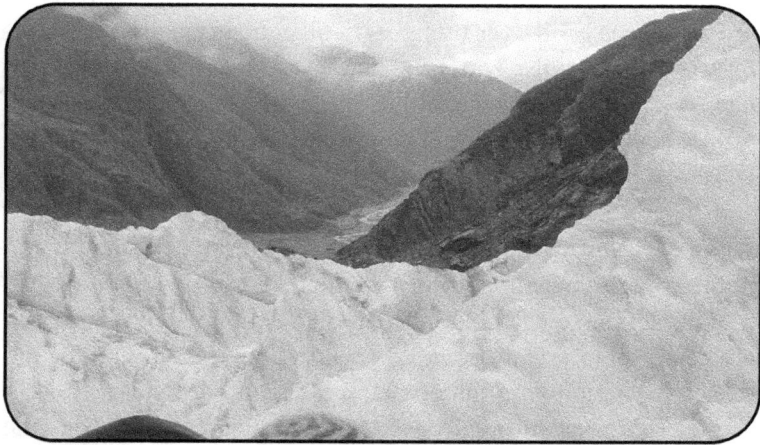

10

Karma

Karma is the tenth Principle of Light and is the second of the higher vibration Principles.

Karma is the balance of energies created by the universe to ensure that every action has its perfect reaction to measure equality and harmony in the flow of life.

Karma balances peace between energies as yin and yang create unity. Karma is a spiritual law that runs through everything we do in life. Karma ensures that what we sow, so shall we reap, and what goes around will always come around. This works for us in both positive and negative ways – if we work at something with heart and muster, doing the best we can, we will receive in equal measure in countless ways. On the other hand, if we treat someone badly or carry out misdeeds over time, these lessons will inevitably come back to haunt us so we might learn from our mistakes.

Karma may roll over lifetimes as all actions are accounted for by individual souls. Karma teaches you how to love, how to understand yourself and how to measure your actions and the effect they have on others. If you learn from karma and heed the lessons it gives you, it will eventually lead you to greater peace and happiness as you move past the projections we all carry within us. You will be able to relate in a more honourable and noble way to your intimates as well as your fellow man.

Our actions connect us to each other in a hidden matrix; we create a ripple effect around us with our thoughts, words and deeds. No action goes unnoticed in the grand design.

Selfless commitment to others and to spirit is the philosophical core of Karma; by benefiting others and the world at large you are welcoming the entry of peace and harmony into your own life.

Karma believes in brotherhood, in working towards a common goal, in helping each other out so that we may all prosper and carry the universal energy pattern forwards into a dimension of higher vibrational existence.

Why Karma is Important

Karma is the great teacher of existence and is beautiful in the precision and accuracy that our life lessons are meted out. There is a harmony and magic in the way we find things coming back to us; there is a synchronicity in the way our challenges are delivered to us, to enable us to grow through both joy and suffering. What we cannot understand now often becomes strikingly clear as time elapses and we look back and see how much we grew in a difficult time, what we learnt from it and how it has added to our current state of awareness and happiness. We are all children on our journey into light, we will all make mistakes along the way and often we will hurt each other. Instead of seeking revenge or hanging onto these hurts it is more important to let go and continue moving, instead of being tied to people and places in the past.

Karma will exact the learning necessary so that others may realize from their transgressions, just as we are dealt certain fates depending on how we treat each other. We must make mistakes in order to learn from them.

Karma initiates us in the rites of spiritual law as we transgress against it. A mark against a fellow man will find its way back to us, and we can either act in righteous indignation, or fully appreciate the taste of our own medicine.

From here, it is our choice to learn the lesson and move forward with forgiveness, or choose to learn it again.

I also believe that karma transcends lifetimes. The concept of reincarnation is supported by several religious belief systems. To believe in reincarnation is to believe in the continuation of life past the flesh, in the journey of the individual spirit through many incarnations, where it continues to amass information, develop through karma and bring this learning to each successive rebirth.

This also sets us free from the pressure to push through everything in one life, and takes away from the sense of failure we may feel if we do not achieve everything in the years allotted to us; we will live to breathe again. It explains the deep subconscious connections we have with others when we feel we may know them instantly and cosmically – it warns that if we act with disrespect and dishonour to the universal energy we may reap the same in another lifetime. People do not get away with great crimes to humanity, even though it appears so in a single incarnation. These beliefs are controversial to some, but in my heart I believe karma works in this way.

Karma is essential in our soul's development over many lifetimes, and with each incarnation, as long as we heed our education, we will become wiser and deeper and broader in our comprehension of our world and our ability to love the people in it. We become more refined, more sensitive and increasingly aware of the effect we have on others – we are less able to separate ourselves from the lives of others or to inflict unjust punishment or cruelty.

We know this because at some stage we have probably lived through it, felt how much it hurts to suffer and are adamant that we will live lives of goodness and peace.

Revenge is a very human condition. When we are wronged by another, we may feel justified in acting out and dealing our own blows to those who have hurt us. We are positively entitled to stand up for ourselves and speak our truth, but calculated revenge is heartless and detracts from our positive flow as it reduces our overall vibration from one of love. To inflict hate on another is to take away from our own state of love – it is far better to release any ties we have to our transgressor and move on in the knowledge that karma will act for us, will teach its own lessons in its own way. We must take a deep breath, have faith in this and turn the other cheek. Two wrongs do not make a right. Karma will educate with compassion and prevent you from harming yourself further by committing your own transgression. People will always make mistakes, people will collide with each other and trip each other up – try to remember that we are all learning and for your own sake let go and move on. Maintain an open loving heart and in your wisdom try not to take things personally. We are all reflecting our inner selves on each other and learning from it. Our greatest challengers in this life are often our wisest teachers. Thank them for what they show you about yourselves, and the love they bring into your life, should you learn from them.

Working with Karma

Answer these questions honestly:

~ Are you aware of karma in your life?
~ Do you give out positive or negative energy to others?
~ Are you currently struggling with challenges in your life?
~ What may your challenges be trying to teach you?
~ Are you aware of your soul purpose and mission?
~ How is karma carrying you closer to your essence?

~ Do you still have negative energies to clear?
~ How could you work to clear these energies and accelerate your journey?
~ Do you believe in reincarnation and past lives?
~ If you do, what wisdom do you think came with you into your current incarnation? Are there any old lessons you may be working through in this lifetime that you need to clear?

Practising Karma

Clearing Past Life Energies

Clearing the karmic record is one way of clearing any old bonds of duty, chastity, poverty and pain that may be holding you back in this lifetime. Your subconscious carries forward old messages from previous lives and you should wipe the slate clean as you work to progress in your current incarnation.

State clearly to the universe and your subconscious:

'I choose to clear my karmic record now so I may work to clear any negative karma in this lifetime and step into my powerful potential as I journey into light.'

Repeat this statement seven times each month for seven months. It is important that the promises you may have made in the past do not slow you down in your current lifetime.

You may find positive energy miraculously flooding into your life as energetic vows are broken and you are free to embrace your current incarnation.

Remedy Store

Flower essences
~ Angelsword (Australian Bush Flower) accessing gifts from past lifetimes and spiritual communication.
~ Boab (Australian Bush Flower) personal freedom from clearing negative karmic and family patterns.

Map your Life History

Write out a history of your life. Include details of your family, early experiences, relationships, education, jobs and significant people and events in your life.

~   What did they teach you; how did they shape you?
~   What did you grow up knowing?
~   What kind of child were you?
~   What kind of person has your life plan made you?
~   Where do you think your natural abilities are best placed?
~   What are you here to do?

Karma in Action

Watch closely and see if you can notice karma in action in your own life, or for those around you. Can you see it working like a hidden magic in every action around you?

Once you have discovered it, it is like opening the door to a secret garden where the answers to life are hidden. Pay attention; learn to trust in the intrinsic synchronicity of karma. Let go of fear, worry and distrust, and find joy and faith in the mastery of spiritual power in everyday life.

Karma and World Power

For every action there is a reaction.

In the current state of world politics, there still exists a great deal of fear, pain and aggression. Man as a global power is struggling to let go of revenge and war. Mother Nature is still under attack, and the energies of our cosmos are in constant turmoil as they try to harmonize beyond the frailty and weakness of mankind. The destruction of our environment continues; our environment will fight back. There is war between many factions of our civilization, and suppression of a minority will lead to a backlash of anger. This cannot continue indefinitely and can only lead to further pain.

I have faith that, eventually, we find peace and learn to cherish what we have been given, but to some, this is a pipe dream – they are still learning, they cannot see, they still make mistakes. We must find compassion for them as they dwell in pain, and hope that karma will duly educate them – meanwhile, we must pray for the safety and sanctity of our universe and promise to lead our own lives by right action and do unto others as we would be done by. If you can do this it will be one small step for mankind and a progression of positive world karma.

Living a Karmic Life

Karma relates to the higher energies in the seventh layer and beyond. The notion of karma is aligned with spiritual law and is therefore channelled through divinity. We receive guidance and reckoning from the in pouring of light, and our own guides and angelic entities will be there to protect us and oversee as we learn from our mistakes and receive blessings from heaven. As we become lighter and freer, we are more able to tune into this frequency and see that there is very little coincidence in life as we approach enlightenment – everything happens for a reason.

Clearing the negative energies from our own matrix accelerates our journey and we move quickly to our rightful place on earth without struggle or suffering. Negativity and wrong action slow us down – if we accept karmic education and agree to repent for our transgressions through learning and love we are able to move beyond our past and into the light. You may notice after a particularly heavy stage where you are dealt challenge after challenge, that if you succeed in rising above matters and maturing in love and wisdom, things will get easier and your rewards will finally flow in. But as in all things, patience and acceptance of flow come first and foremost. The universe will only deliver complete happiness when you know what it means, appreciate it justly, protect it in good measure and won't risk it by doing wrong to another.

We struggle to learn humility and compassion. As immature souls we are blinkered to the realities in others' lives and are intrinsically selfish. The ego says 'me first' and we obey its commands. We may run riot over others' sensitivities and pursue a life of transgressions accumulating on weak foundations. With karma to guide us we will learn that there is greater joy to be found by sharing our blessings and goodness, loving each other, showing compassion to the vulnerable and weak and living by a code of honour. This submission to spiritual law over the material brings us great understanding and scope in our ability to carry ourselves, bring happiness to others and continually find joy in the beauty and wonder of everyday life and the miracles in the hidden workings of the world we live in. This opening and amazement at seeing beyond the primary dimension of life and watching karma in action is often enough to renew your faith in the universe and deepen your enjoyment of your own existence. The world takes on new meaning. The joy of being selfish is overrun by the selfish joy of being kind and considerate, as the overwhelming good feeling it generates gives you a warm glow that is greater than any pain associated from taking from another.

Goodwill comes back to you and bathes your existence in a golden light.

Watching karma and the grand design allows you to piece together the events and moments in your life and see a thread, common themes, significant events, a mission and a truth. Nothing is a coincidence. Once you can perceive in this manner it is easier to let go of sorrow and regret, bitterness and shame, and begin to live in your entirety as you realize everything is moving you closer to a common goal. You are here to learn and grow and fulfil your soul purpose. Look at your life in this way and see the divine plan for the first time. Honour the essence that was carried through with you at your birth and have faith in karma that it will continue to move you effortlessly closer to this point with peace and happiness.

~   Karma is a measure of your earthly experiences.
~   Karma harmonizes, regulates and instructs wisely.
~   Karma transcends all energies.
~   Karma delivers justice.

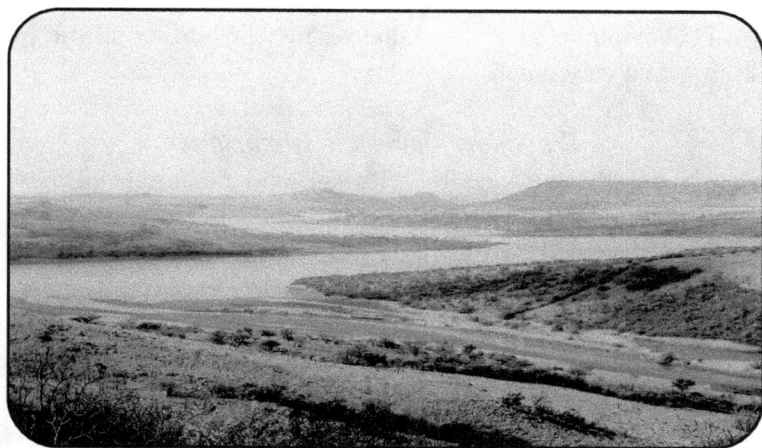

11

Forgiveness

Forgiveness is the eleventh Principle of Light and is the third of our higher vibration collective.

Forgiveness speaks of true compassion, love and understanding and the milk of human kindness. Forgiveness is powerful and perceptive, all-knowing and wise, and sees through human weakness by turning the other cheek and giving and feeling love, even in times of great adversity.

Forgiveness is truly the greatest human challenge, for how do we teach ourselves to love when we have been deeply hurt or let down? How is this even possible?

But we have all seen the act of forgiveness in motion and felt its tenderness and power. We have all been blessed by the hand of forgiveness, and have moved on to live another day.

We can all appreciate how freeing it is to be forgiven for our mistakes, although most of the time we cannot see through our own behaviour or understand that we may be hurting people we in fact love very much.

Why Forgiveness is Important

Forgiveness comes easily with an understanding of how important karma is in our lives. If Karma is the Principle of spiritual education, and learning from our mistakes, forgiveness is the oil in the wheels that allows us to keep moving and growing beyond them. If we are wronged we will try to allow for another's false actions towards us, express our feelings and regret in truth, but then allow that person to move on by letting go. We may not be able to grow with that person in our lives anymore but this does not prevent us from deep forgiveness. We trust that karma will support us if we learn from our part in the interaction, and will seek to educate our transgressor. We will learn how to defend and protect ourselves in the future and we know that karma will take care of the rest. We fill our hearts with love and find peace again.

If we hold anger and resentment at the moment when the other person's transgression occurred, we remain rooted to that point in time and bound to the person whose actions have let us down. We may think to ourselves that if we stop harbouring a grudge we will be letting that person 'get away with it'. In fact, what actually happens is that we weigh ourselves down with our hatred and bitterness and pollute our own hearts with vibrations other than love. The fury and negativity will burn away at our own heart energy and in fact have much less impact on the person that we are angry at. The act of blaming someone else for our continuing pain detracts from our own ability to change our circumstances; if we feel our happiness is dependent on another person we diminish our own transition by refusing complete responsibility for what is happening now.

In energetic terms forgiveness becomes quite a selfish act; the forgiveness benefits us more than anyone, as it relinquishes the carriage of darker energies that may harm us and become buried in our psyche or physical bodies, causing stress and ill health.

So the most powerful act of love we can give ourselves is to forgive those whose deeds have hurt us and forgive ourselves for our own mistakes and wrong action. We are only human and we are only learning; the majority of wrongdoing originates from ignorance, poor communication, fear and sadness. As children we find it easy to forgive; we seem to know only how to love. We would rather experience joy and adventure than pain and regret. We do not yet understand guilt or shame and generally find it easy to express our anger or pain immediately and then move on.

As children we have not developed the ability to mask our inner feelings of disappointment or betrayal, however trivial it may seem, but express freely. The mask we wear as adults means we can hide our less socially acceptable feelings from others but by doing so we also opt to hide them from ourselves. The healthy way to deal with anger and frustration is to acknowledge it to ourselves and pay it respect as we feel it. If we own up to being let down, upset or hurt we can then deal with it accordingly, instead of burying it in our subconscious and letting it brew and stew, until it takes on a life of its own. We may choose to confront the person who has hurt us in an honest and constructive way, rather than blow up or become aggressive at a later stage; this way we defend our own rights and make our point heard.

Once we have expressed our feelings honestly and know we have been heard it becomes easier to forgive. Once we have both agreed to let bygones be bygones and walk forwards into a new future with a better understanding of each other it is worthwhile to forgive. Once forgiveness of others becomes easy we find it far easier to forgive ourselves for the mistakes we have made.

We can start again, living today, living in the present.

Forgive and ye shall be blessed.

Working with Forgiveness

Answer these questions honestly:

~ Who do you need to forgive?
~ Why?
~ Do you feel you can forgive?
~ If not, why not?
~ Are you willing to try?
~ Are there any reasons you do not want to let go?
~ Do you need to forgive yourself for anything?
~ Do you feel yourself capable of finding unconditional love above all else?
~ What transgressions are easy to forgive and which are not?
~ What does forgiveness mean to you and how could you make this a bigger part of your life?

Practising Forgiveness

Letting Go

Finding true forgiveness takes time. If you feel there are major blocks standing in your way or you are resisting healing, start by affirming seven times, morning and night: 'I am willing to forgive and set myself free.'

Do not worry if you cannot imagine forgiving people who have caused you great harm at this stage.

Sometimes, it is first necessary to be angry and allow yourself to feel this emotion without any denial. Be angry; write about it, talk about it, let the feelings rise and then let them go. Once you respect your own feelings and allow this to happen naturally it is simpler to release from the past and move away from what has hurt you. This detachment enables inflowing compassion towards your transgressor and starts the healing process.

Focus on your own willingness to let go of the past and move forward; concentrate on letting the light in so you may be healed.

Visualization to Clear the Heart

Imagine a white light channelling from your crown, flooding your heart and cleansing the space of any negative energies.

Focus especially on removing guilt, resentment, bitterness and blame.

If you are ready to forgive others in your past take this time to visualize them from a safe place; cut any cords that may be binding you still to them, grant them love and forgiveness and request that they now leave your field.

Allow your guides and angels to assist you in this, all the while reciting your affirmation: 'I am willing to forgive.'

Sit in peace for five to ten minutes every day, allowing this pure energy to enter your consciousness.

Imagine you are forgiving yourself and others for any blame or bitterness you have been carrying; forgive those others in the world who have caused harm and destruction to humanity. We all need forgiveness to grow.

Looking Back on Your Past

Look back on your past and remember times when you were hurt, saddened, betrayed or injured. What has happened to these memories? Can you look back with a smile on your face or do they still hurt? How did you deal with the pain? Do these incidents need healing? Are you still angry with certain people in your past?

If you have moved on you will find looking back is easy and what was very painful at the time has now receded into the distance. You may find yourself able to laugh or smile at something that was once very painful. If you still feel anger, anxiety or tension remembering certain things you may need to work on forgiveness with the people involved, or forgive yourself if you feel you made mistakes. You may still be harbouring feelings of rage or frustration towards those others or yourself. These 'mistakes' may have been actions that were entirely necessary, and continuing to blame sets you back. Have you ever let anyone down in your life because you had to or you didn't know how to do things better. I'm sure you have, so forgive others as you forgive yourself.

Use imagery and visualization to cut any ties to people in your past and send love to the parts of yourself that deserve attention.

Learn to let go; it is time to step forward into your future.

Forgiveness in Everyday Life

Practise everyday forgiveness and try to look through people's mistakes as they make them. Protect yourself and try not to take it personally. You will find it a lot easier to cleanse guilt and self-blame from your own heart and those around you will show you increasing compassion by the Principle of karma in action.

Remedy Store

Flower essences

~ Holly (Bach) releases hatred.
~ Dagger Hakea (Australian Bush Flower) releases resentment and bitterness.
~ Staphysagria (homeopathic remedy) for suppressed anger.

Living a Forgiving Life

Forgiveness is not about becoming a victim.

You may feel that by letting go you have been walked over. You may think that by failing to seek revenge you are being weak.

Power and strength are open-minded, truthful and protective. It is right and correct to stand up for yourself and allow your voice to be heard. It is foolish to attract danger to your path. It is wise and magnanimous to see beyond another's wrong actions and find compassion in your heart. It is right to trust the universe. It is kind and loving to keep your heart open and empty of hatred.

Let go of your anger and forgive. Do not allow your soul to sink down but rise up. Believe in your own greatness and do not dwell on the small upsets that fall in your path. Step up and over them and leave flowers in your wake, as you move ever closer to the light.

Revenge can sometimes seem like the only action available. If someone hurts you or your loved ones your first instinct in your anger and distress is to fight back and hurt in equal measure. In the case of physical self-defence this may be necessary but often we feel the need to punish or reduce after we have been emotionally wounded. We may plot and plan, scheme and manipulate, our resentment growing like a cold, dark corner in our soul. This is heart blindness, madness, and such a course of action may often lead to further ruin for us. Two wrongs do not make a right. If we allow ourselves that time to calm down, still ourselves and move past our initial shock our choices may be quite different. Forgiveness does not mean that we need to hold those who hurt us close; in many cases it is better to move to new pastures and give ourselves the time and space to heal fully. Forgiveness is about turning our lives around after a difficult experience, realizing that every soul is on a journey and occasionally we all take a fall.

How easy is it to forgive? I would say at times it is the most impossible thing on earth and at others it is simple. We can forgive a child who breaks something in an instant as we accept their vulnerability and youth. The stranger who comes out of the blue to assault us or steal from us is another matter. How can you forgive something so wicked? How could you find forgiveness for a murderer, a rapist or a terrorist?

It may seem impossible. It may never happen. We may never find that gentleness in our lives to do so again.

But at some stage, we may try to forgive, after many years, as forgiveness is the final piece in our healing. It is the last piece of jigsaw that clicks into place with the healing of our heart and our readiness to live life in its fullest, without fear. We are able to see our aggressor as an expression of human suffering and let go of any hatred that we may hold for that person.

It is wise to acknowledge that there are those who lose their way and innocent lives are affected in the process, but continuing to hate does not stop this happening, and only reduces the lives we have.

Life is a gift to be cherished. In the process of healing there is an important fact to remember. Forgiveness cannot be forced. If something terrible does happen to you, forgiveness may never come. This is something you need to forgive yourself for.

If you try to rush the process and offer false forgiveness because this is the right thing to do and all the books tell you to, it will not ring true.

You have to feel forgiveness in your bones. Also, trying to forgive injustice is very hard to comprehend at stage one of the healing process and does not feel natural; it should never be expected and the phrase should be 'you don't have to forgive – only if you want to.' This allows the soul the freedom to move through different emotions easily and healthily, one by one. We have no comprehension at stage one how we will feel at stage five and nor should we. A journey is valid because of the route we take and not because we leap forwards to the destination.

We must first find acknowledgement, anger, betrayal, sadness, grief and acceptance before we even begin to touch on compassion and forgiveness. We need to expunge the heavy energies from our heart before we can rise again to the vibration of unconditional love for humanity. Each person will take their own time in this depending on their personality type, the nature of the insult and their general vitality and willingness to heal.

Forgiveness allows us to look back on our past as a history. It makes short stories of the ups and downs of our lives that we can look at with fondness; we can see how we have grown through adversity and realize the depth of our joy compared to the feelings of sadness. It allows us to look back and see the river running – we have no desire to remain in an unhappy past, we should hope that we are always carried to a more joyful future.

Forgiveness and detachment permit reasoning and compassion. Forgiveness puts sadness in perspective; a contour in our otherwise happy lives. Forgiveness leaves the things that didn't work so well as memories of our youth. Forgiveness makes us realize that our greatest challenges in life, and the people that bring them, are our greatest teachers. If we choose to hold onto bitterness we cannot make that step into the future; we cannot empty ourselves of pain and fill up again with love, we are forever tied to our bad memories and our tragedies and we allow them to dwarf our vision. Forgiveness sets the past free and puts us firmly in the present.

Who do you need to forgive? Forgiveness directed at the self is often forgotten. Do we even appreciate how much we blame ourselves for making mistakes, letting people down, not being good enough or perfect enough? Do we neglect the inner child that deserves respect and unconditional love in all of us and continually come down too hard?

It is especially important to free your own heart from guilt and stop punishing yourself for things you feel you could have done better or differently. Directing anger towards your own energy body has the same effect as being angry with others, and corrodes the gentle heart. If you feel you deserve blame and punishment you will attract situations or people to you who make you feel this way, to reiterate the feeling of low self-worth you carry inside. You take the role of a victim, allowing others to hurt you.

There may be reasons you do not want to let go of your negative emotions. As long as they reside inside you they eat up valuable energy, stop you believing in yourself and loving yourself fully and stand in the way of achieving your true potential. They may provide a safety net when things become too good; they provide a point of reference and a reminder that happiness is fallible.

Are you too afraid to find peace and the joy of living you deserve? You do not deserve blame or hardship. You deserve compassion and forgiveness. You deserve love and happiness.

If you need to make amends or right your wrongs, do so and then let go. Allow karma to direct your actions but do not feel karma will give you more than you can handle.

Do not fear karma as a disciplinarian who will seek revenge; karma is born of love and wisdom. Forgive your inner child and find love again. You did what you needed to do with the information you had at the time; this is the same for everyone on their path into light, they are doing the best they can.

Try not to take things too personally; remember, angels fly lightly for a reason. Forgiveness is the final step in the search for salvation. For our universe to understand and for us to work with forgiveness is to accept and forgive the sins of our fathers and move forwards as a unified force into a brave new world.

Forgiveness

~   Forgiveness demands a fine and pure spiritual vibration to descend throughout our universe.
~   Forgiveness is the greatest act that mankind can make – love in the face of loss and destruction.
~   Forgiveness believes in love and believes that man is making this transition.
~   Forgiveness believes in a better future for everyone.
~   I forgive you and I set you free with love.
~   Forgiveness is the key that opens the door to divine light.

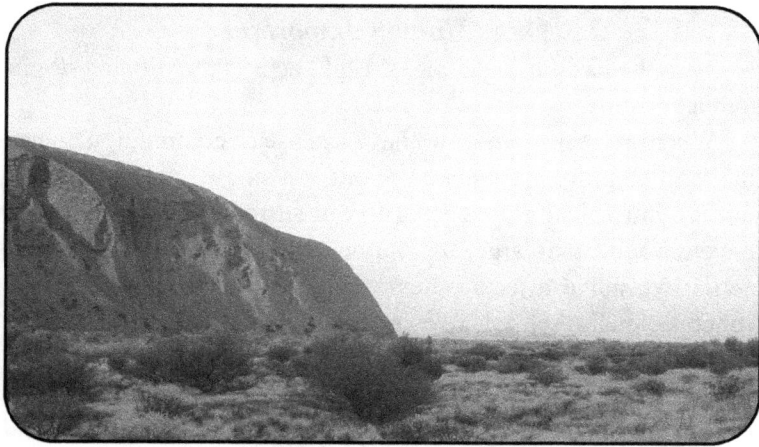

12

Unity

Unity is the harmonic Principle of love, integration and complete connection. Unity is the Principle that binds us together, that makes no difference between us, that believes we all came from the same place, we all have the same race; the brotherhood of man.

We stand as one and as one we go forth into the world we are building for ourselves. We all play a part in the history of our universe and we all are responsible for our future here on earth. As a united force we have power; power to change for the good, power to create miracles, power to transcend our human limitations and walk the rest of our days in peace.

Unity speaks of the golden land where our descendants can rest in the days that are fruits of our labours now. Unity makes everything possible.

Why Unity is Important

Unity is the twelfth Principle of Light as it is the nirvana of our human destiny.

When we realize unity we have a sense of communion, hence the term community. We are no longer a single, isolated energy, but are intrinsically connected to our surroundings, each other, the environment at large, and our universe. We can see that every action we make affects others, that every thought we have is subconsciously sensed. We are all part of the same matrix, energetically connected by invisible but tangible threads of life, binding our fates together. Man is not an island; he may shape his life but in doing so separates himself from all the wonder and joy to be found by learning from each other and loving each other.

Mankind is just one expression of the life force, along with the birds, the trees, the oceans, and the mountains. Life force is ever-present and spreads her bounty into myriad dimensions and expressions of beauty. Who can fail to be amazed by the little miracles they witness each day; if you have ever seen a child born this is true affirmation that life is beautiful and will continue to be so, as long as we respect and appreciate all that we have been given.

Every shade of life, every nuance, every wild and diverse imagination is present; all derived from a single point. We are all expressions of the same force, all mirroring each other and bringing forth a tiny fraction of a greater power. If we look at the world in this way it is hard not to see the greater unity. If we look at our universe from a distant point, we are all one – struggling and fighting and living and breathing, experiencing pain and having fun and sharing moments of tenderness.

You see, we all feel the same things.

If you have ever done group work or have met a collection of strangers and got to know them a little better you will be amazed by the fact that they are similar to you, not different, if you scratch beneath the surface. Getting to know different types of people from different walks of life, I continue to find that we all carry secret pain which we are too scared to share, we all have had times where we feel lonely, lost and confused, that we are equally hoping to have a life in which we can love and be loved and find a way to make things happier and easier. Realizing these similarities brings us closer; we are more able to comfort each other, we feel less burdened by our stories and are wiser for knowing that there are others who have walked our path and made it through the wilderness.

There is hope.

We need to embody that sense in ourselves, a sense of togetherness; we are not the only ones who suffer, we are not the only ones who feel pain. Look around you at all those people out there who we judge on a daily basis – they each have their story and they are all dealing with their lives in their own way. Don't believe everything you see or assume, think deeper and look for the inner child in everyone. Try not to blame but try to understand. Don't stand back and take judgement, look closer and think hard. Do you really know what that person across from you is feeling, thinking, doing; do you know what has happened on his path?

He may be a lot like you inside, despite his colour, creed, position in society, age or sex. Look to the heart of the person and remember to think and do as you would be done by – we are all part of the same energy; wherever we come from, we are all on the same journey, we are all one.

Working with Unity

Answer these questions honestly:
~ Do you feel unified in your mind, body and soul?
~ Do you feel connected with others in your world?
~ Do you have a sense of community?
~ If not, how could you improve this?
~ Do you carry any prejudice towards other cultures or belief systems?

~   If so, why do you think this is?
~   How does it affect your own heart energy to feel this way?
~   Can you forgive others completely in order to attain unity?
~   Do you sense a primal connection to mankind?
~   Do you see the world as One World, or a group of countries, each with their own agenda?

Practising Unity

Visualisation to Achieve Unity
~   Harmonize your complete energy field and allow divine light to flood your consciousness.
~   Submit to the incoming vibration and accept the high-level frequency of divine light.
~   Fall to spiritual bliss and rise up, lift your vibration to a superluminal consciousness where we are all light energy, connected by spiritual love.

Use this visualization every night while meditating; ask the light to unify your entire energy field and guide you to a greater sense of harmony.

Community
Work with your own sense of community and think of this as a much larger space than you are used to.

Think of ways you could improve the lives of others in your world, even if the action is small. Could you start recycling, donate to a local charity or perhaps give your time to help another person in your community.

Many small actions make a great one. One person is all it takes to change the world.

Recognition Exercise

Next time you interact with someone you do not know so well, see if you can look into their eyes more deeply than you would normally.

What can you see? Do you simply see his face or can you see sparkle, intellect, a fire dancing or life energy? Can you see spirit? Can you see a connection? When you look into the eyes of people from different walks of life, different countries, different races, are they really so different to you? The eyes are the windows to the soul – we all have a collective soul.

See if you can see your face in the mirror.

Remedy Store

~ Sydney Rose (Australian Bush Flower) realising we are all one.

Living a Unified Life

Unity seeks community. Unity calls for integration. Unity asks that we make connections. Unity asks that we become more efficient, more powerful and more aware of each other. Unity demands that we find harmony and balance within the self. Unity makes us understand that by working with one another we become less alone. Unity creates energy from health. Unity takes pride in what we have been given in life and strives to make it even better. Unity takes responsibility for the less able in our world; and so the strong shall help the weak. Unity calls for brotherhood and hope.

Much of the devastation and destruction in our world comes from a separatist consciousness; where man is not big enough to see beyond his own doorstep. Separatism cannot look into another man's eyes and see a similarity or a likeness; what it sees is something he can hold up as different and foreign.

Ignorance and contempt breed hatred. What man often finds most difficult to deal with is the shadow that lives within. He seeks to destroy what he cannot abide in others, as he has not found what he unconditionally loves in himself.

He sees the alien other as something quite distant from himself, he cannot respond to the integral bonds of humanity; this prevents him from feeling and acting in a humane manner.

When we are unified we do not see the 'us and them'. We see that to give and love others is to give and love ourselves and our own; we see harming or hurting another man as something we must reckon with in our own heart and conscience.

We have unification and harmony of the mind, body and soul. Our own self-integration is reflected in the healthy view we uphold of the others in our universe.

By disconnecting our emotions and soul we are able to treat our fellow man clinically, mechanically. We can see them as statistics and numbers. It enables us to think rationally and logically. It allows us to inflict harm, carry out atrocities.

The people in faraway lands who live through war, lose their children and homes and harbour the tragedy of crisis for decades afterwards, are in truth our responsibility. The sooner we face this fact and reconnect our hearts with our brains, the sooner we will find salvation and peace. There are many of us lucky enough to have been born in a safe, stable country, where we are clothed, sheltered, educated and fed. It is our duty as a world power to seek unity instead of continuing to support separation.

When we separate from others we forget that they too have feelings, emotions and sensitivities. We judge the exterior and make comparisons with what we perceive on the outside. We project our own insecurities and shadow onto another person and if we find we do not like what we see we withdraw our love. In this instant we are creating a little less love for ourselves. We may be jealous of someone, from what we hear or see, or we may take offence at the way a person behaves or what they say. If we have a strong reaction we are reacting to our own projections, rather than simply observing a course of events. We may decide we do not like this person as they make us feel bad about ourselves, and instead of looking within we send out fear and hatred and pull ourselves away. By doing this we are pulling away from communing, from unity.

We should focus inwards when situations make us uncomfortable, examine our own weakness and find out how to heal these areas. Finding fault with others is no solution and casting blame is an excuse for not taking personal responsibility.

Separatism takes from love and leads to loneliness and isolation. Unity asks for love and connection in all places. Our hearts beat together. We are born, live and die together. We sing and dance and smile together. We learn from each other and teach each other. We find courage in our hearts to perform miracles that bring us closer. We all want to live in a peaceful world where our children are safe.

We extend a hand to those who ask for our help. We fight each other and we seek each other's forgiveness. We love each other.

For all this we must remember we share our lives. We could not exist if it were not for those souls around us, or find the breath to experience joy or pain. Our lives would have little meaning if it were not for the others who share our universe.

Appreciate every single one of them right now, the ones you love, the ones you don't know and especially the ones you hate, for they are teaching you what you need to learn to grow.

Unity

~ We are one.

~ You and I live together.

~ My heart goes out to you and my love will be eternal in this world.

~ Unity is the grail at the end of the journey into light.

~ Unity is enlightenment.

~ Unity is the end that our souls yearn for; perfect bliss.

~ Unity is sensing the vibration above pain, where we can exist in the ether, rising above man's imperfections.

~ Unity unites us with every molecule in the cosmos and makes us a small part of that energy.

~ The ego is left behind for the higher reaches of pure soul consciousness and we see beyond the limitations of a material incarnation.

~ Unity is free spirit.

~ Unity forgives the transgressions of mankind as it sees those actions as part of the global soul advancement.

~ Unity is willing to forgive completely so we can all move on together with love in our hearts.

~ Unity is forever bringing us closer together instead of further apart.

~ Unity looks at each part of our universe as a perfect representation of the total picture. Each universe is represented in one man, a journey waiting to be discovered.

~ Unity is holographic.

~ Unity brings elevation of the human race to the wonderment of heaven and its pure and beautiful vibrations as we love and accept each other deeply.

~ Unity knows no bounds and may defeat all obstacles in its quest for the truth.

~ Unity lives in the freedom of soul harmony.

Epilogue

Thank you for taking this journey with me.

It has offered me challenges, insights and unutterable joy along the way. I hope you find the same sense of wonder that I have, as I found the words to express my innermost dreams, hopes and desires for our planet.

The Journey into Light is an eternal path that we travel over lifetimes, and I am truly looking forward to the winding road ahead.

Our world is truly beautiful and I am honoured to have the opportunity to adventure through her lands.

To all Spirits, rejoice in the good times ahead of us, and keep learning and loving and laughing.

May the universe be with you in every step that you take.

Appendix

Safe Essential Oils to Use During Pregnancy
Benzoin
Bergamot
Grapefruit
Lavender
Lemon
Neroli
Orange
Patchouli
Sandalwood
Spearmint
Tea Tree
Vetiver

It is advisable to contact a qualified practitioner to work with you if you would like to try aromatherapy massage, as each woman is individual in her health needs during pregnancy. Otherwise, it is safe to add a few drops to your bath or pillow.

Working with Crystals

Crystals have intelligent energy which, when utilized successfully, can transform our own vibrations with their fine frequencies. To work with them it is essential that they are cleaned and prepared first to remove any existing stagnant energy.

Clean them with water, visualizing the dirty energy washing away.

If you have time, it is preferable to soak them in salt water overnight prior to cleaning.

Use incense or your own energy to cleanse any lingering physical or psychic energy from the crystals.

Leave them in sunlight or moonlight to charge for up to 24 hours.

Ask for divine blessing and instruct the crystal to heal you in whichever way you need.

Leave the crystal by your bed to work its magic overnight, wear it or place it for periods of time over a blocked chakra.

Do not use crystal healing during pregnancy.

List of
Therapists and Resources

NHS General Practitioners
Patient resource at www.rcgp.org.uk is Patient Centre - How to use your GP/surgery. GPs can make an assessment and refer you to specialist practitioners as required or advise you on the best course of action to take. They are the gateway to the NHS service and can refer you to psychiatry and psychology services.

British Association of Psychotherapists
37 Mapesbury Road
London NW2 4HJ
0208 452 9823
www.bap-psychotherapy.org
This register should point you to a therapist in your area.

British Homeopathic Association
www.trusthomeopathy.org
info@trusthomeopathy.org
0870 444 3950
The BHA can give you advice about using homeopathy and finding a practitioner.

British Acupuncture Council
www.acupuncture.org.uk
info@acupuncture.org.uk

0208 735 0400
The BAC can give you a list of qualified acupuncturists in your area.

National Institute of Medical Herbalists
www.nimh.org.uk
nimh@exeter.freeserve.co.uk
01392 426022
Contact for registered herbalists in your area.

Aromatherapy Organisations Council
www.aromatherapy-regulation.org.uk
info@aromatherapy-regulation.org.uk
0870 7743 477
Contact for registered practitioners in your area.

The Hale Clinic
7 Park Crescent, London W1B 1PF
Tel: 020 7631 0156   Fax: 020 7580 5771
www.haleclinic.com
info@haleclinic.com
Dr. Millie Saha practises Fusion Medicine at the Hale Clinic; contact details shown above.

The Hypnotherapy Association
www.thehypnotherapyassociation.co.uk
admin@thehypnotherapyassociation.co.uk
01257 262124
Association of professional psychotherapists using hypnotherapy to resolve emotional issues.

British Reflexology Association
www.britflex.cco.uk
bra@britreflex.co.uk
01886 821207
Contact for more about reflexology and local practitioners.

The British Wheel Of Yoga
www.bwy.org.uk
office@bwy.org.uk
01529 306 851
Lists teachers trained in all schools of yoga therapy.

General Osteopathic Council
www.osteopathy.org.uk
info@osteopathy.org.uk
0207 357 6655
If you have problems with posture, back or hip pain, contact a
therapist on the national register.

The British Naturopathic Association
www.naturopaths.co.uk
0870 745 6984
Your local naturopath can provide natural, gentle healthcare.

British Nutrition Foundation
www.nutrition.org.uk
Links to finding a registered nutritionist in your area.

The Reiki Association
www.reikiassociation.org.uk
co-ordinator@reikiassociation.org.uk
0901 8800 009
Lists registered reiki practitioners in your area.

Bach Flower Essences
www.bachcentre.com
Find out more about the essences and how they can heal you.

The Association for Meridian Energy Therapies
www.theamt.com
The register of AMT practitioners and resources.

Kinesiology Federation
www.kinesiologyfederation.org
Register of kinesiologists, and lots of information about the therapy.

Pranic Healing International
www.pranichealing.org
Resource site for pranic healing.

Institute of Complementary Medicine
www.icmedicine.co.uk
icm@icmedicine.co.uk
0207 237 5165
Information on complementary medicine and how to find a registered practitioner.

Prince of Wales Foundation for Integrated Health
www.fihealth.org.uk
info@fihealth.org.uk
020 3119 3100
Providing information about the integration of conventional and complementary healthcare.

Index

A
Abundance 35
addiction 58
Addictions, Confront Your 63
Addressing Pain and Trauma 29
alcohol 143
Amethyst 119, 132
Authenticity 78

B
Bach's Flower Essences 119
Benzoin 174
Bergamot 174
Black tourmaline 31

C
caffeine 143
Celestite 119, 132
Chakras, The 9
childhood 25, 53
Clearing Past Life Energies 151
Community 168
concentration 119
cords 31
Creativity 51
Creativity Journal 64
Creativity, Nurture 63

Crystal Therapy 119
Crystals 14, 91, 103, 132

D
Dealing with your Truth 101
drugs 143

E
Essences 14
Essential oils 14, 119, 174

F
fear 80
Fears, Confront Your 78
Flower Essences 91
Fluorite 119
Forgiveness 155

G
Gaia 35
Geranium 119
Giving and Receiving 47
Global Protection 32
Grapefruit 174

H
Harnessing Natural Energy Flow 45
Health 143

Heart, Clear the 159
heavenly wisdom 119
Higher Soul Collective 138
homeopathy 14
How does Abundance
Develop? 37
How does Creativity
Develop? 53
How does Love Develop? 83
How does Protection
Develop? 24
How does Surrender
Develop? 127
How does Trust Develop? 70
How does Truth Develop? 97
How does Wisdom Develop?
109

I
Illness, The Meaning of 7
indecision 119
Integrated Medicine 11

J
Journal Writing 78

K
Karma 147
Karma and World Power 152
Karma in Action 152
Keep a Straight Head 120

L
lapis lazuli 103
Lavender 174
Lemon 174

Listen, Learning to 102
Living a Creative Life 64
Living a Forgiving Life 160
Living a Karmic Life 153
Living a Loving Life 92
Living a Peaceful Life 144
Living a Protected Life 32
Living a Trusting Life 78
Living a Truthful Life 104
Living a Unified Life 169
Living a Wise Life 121
Living an Abundant Life 48
Love 81
Love, Meditate on 90

M
Map your Life History 152
Master's Way 108
memories, hidden 101

N
Neroli 174
Nurture Yourself 91

O
Orange 119, 174

P
Patchouli 174
Peace 139
Peace, Find 142
Positive Intention 30
Positive Thought Power 62
Practice Loving Kindness 92
Practising Abundance 45
Practising Creativity 62

Practising Forgiveness 158
Practising Karma 151
Practising Love 90
Practising Peace 142
Practising Protection 30
Practising Surrender 131
Practising Trust 75
Practising Truth 101
Practising Unity 168
Practising Wisdom 118
Procreation 66
Protection 21
Psychotherapy 121
Purity of Thought 30

Q
Quartz, Clear 119
Quartz, Snowy 132

R
Recognition Exercise 169
Releasing Pain 10
Resources 176
Rosemary 119

S
Sage, Clary 119
Sandalwood 174
Scleranthus 119
Self-Care 46
Sexual Trauma 59
Spearmint 174
spiritual awakening 119
spiritual law 147
Sugar 143
Surrender 125

Surrendering to Life 134
Sydney Rose 169

T
Tea Tree 174
Therapists 176
Thoughts, Check your 118
Trust 67
Truth 95
Truth, Accept the 118
turquoise 103

U
Unity 165
Use your Voice Wisely 102

V
Vetiver 174
Vibrations 8

W
Walnut 31
When Abundance is Strong 39
When Abundance is Weak 41
When Creativity is Strong 55
When Creativity is Weak 56
When Love is Strong 86
When Love is Weak 87
When Protection is Strong 26
When Protection is Weak 27
When Surrender is Strong 129
When Surrender is Weak 130
When Trust is Strong 72
When Trust is Weak 73
When Truth is Strong 98

When Truth is Weak 99
When Wisdom is Strong 112
When Wisdom is Weak 114
Why Abundance is Important 36
Why Creativity is Important 52
Why Forgiveness is Important 156
Why Karma is Important 148
Why Love is Important 82
Why Peace is Important 140
Why Protection is Important 22
Why Surrender is Important 126
Why Trust is Important 68
Why Truth is Important 96
Why Unity is Important 166
Why Wisdom is Important 108
Wild Oat 119
Wisdom 107
Wisdom and the Energy Field 110
Working with Abundance 44
Working with Creativity 61
Working with Crystals 175
Working with Forgiveness 158
Working with Karma 150
Working with Love 89
Working with Peace 141
Working with Protection 28
Working with Surrender 131
Working with Trust 75
Working with Truth 101
Working with Unity 167
Working with Wisdom 117
World Peace 144
Worship the God/Goddess Within 63
Write a Life Plan 142

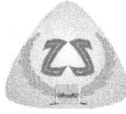

Zambezi Publishing Ltd

We hope you have enjoyed reading this book. The Zambezi range of books includes titles by top level, internationally acknowledged authors on fresh, thought-provoking viewpoints in your favourite subjects. A common thread with all our books is the easy accessibility of content; we have no sleep-inducing tomes, just down-to-earth, easily digestible, credible books.

Please visit our website at www.zampub.coma to browse our full range of Lifestyle and Mind, Body & Spirit titles, and to see what might spark your interest next...

Our books are available from good bookshops throughout the UK; many are available in the USA, sometimes under different titles and ISBNs used by our USA co-publisher, Sterling Publishing Co, Inc.

Please note:-

Nowadays, no bookshop can hope to carry in stock more than a fraction of the books published each year (over 200,000 new titles were published in the UK last year!). However, most UK bookshops can order and supply our titles swiftly, in no more than a few days (within the UK). If they say not, that's incorrect.

You can also find all our books on amazon.co.uk, other UK internet bookshops, and many are also on amazon.com.

Our website (www.zampub.com) also carries and sells our whole range, direct to you.

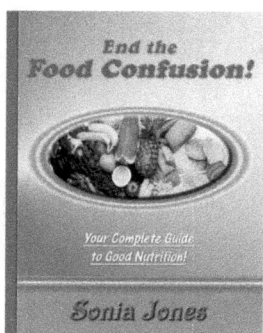

End the Food Confusion

Sonia Jones ND

Nutritional information is often confusing, contradictory, complicated and impractical. Sonia's book takes us through the values and contents of a huge variety of food and vitamins, to show clearly what actually happens to our bodies when we treat them well, or how we damage them by eating badly.

~~~~~~

This book is for everyone, including vegetarians and dieters, with a terrific range of delicious recipes for most requirements. Sonia takes a sensible view of what comprises a balanced and healthy diet, thus allowing us to choose, easily and naturally, the right mix for a healthy, zest-filled lifestyle.

~~~~~~

Sonia Jones is a qualified Naturopath, Dietary Therapist and Reflexologist, with years of experience in Australia, and running her own clinics in the UK and Malta.

She has now achieved her long-standing ambition of creating a first-class clinic in Valle Escondido, a beautiful spot in Panama, where she specialises in chronic illness and holistic diet programs, along with a variety of naturopathic therapies.

ISBN 978-1-903065-72-3   272 pages   RRP £12.99

www.ingramcontent.com/pod-product-compliance
Lightning Source LLC
Chambersburg PA
CBHW072141270326
41931CB00010B/1833